A PRACTICAL
STEP BY STEP GUIDE TO

Full Mouth Reconstruction

FOR GENERAL DENTAL PRACTITIONERS

HOW TO PROGRESS FROM SINGLE TOOTH DENTISTRY TO DIRECT ADHESIVE FULL MOUTH RECONSTRUCTION

Dr. Devang Patel

A Practical Step by Step Guide to Full Mouth Reconstruction
How to Progress from Single Tooth Dentistry to Direct Adhesive Full Mouth Reconstruction
By Dr Devang Patel

Publisher: Addea Media

ISBN 978-1-7399431-2-7

This is a live book. Upon registration at the link provided in the book you will receive regular updates to the information provided within the book.

CONTENTS

Foreword

If you ask me to name a single factor without which my current success would not have been possible, then meeting Dr Devang Patel would be it. I work in a successful private practice carrying out all the treatments that dentistry has to offer from simple treatment such as composite bonding to complex treatment such as full mouth reconstruction and implant placement and bone grafting procedures. This is merely 6 years after I completed my vocational training.

I met Dr Devang Patel when I was looking to find a mentor to improve my dental skills. Devang guided me throughout my dental career and he continues to play a huge role in my progress in dentistry. I met Devang in 2015 when I was doing my vocational training. Within the next four years I progressed under his mentorship from the stage of doing very basic dentistry to providing great dental services to my patients including full mouth reconstructions under the reorganised approach, as well placing and restoring dental implants. Devang is a very passionate, highly skilled dentist who is very logical and great at treatment planning based on the patient's individual needs. His forte in dentistry is complex restorative work including extreme wear cases, implant treatments involving extensive grafting and he consistently achieves amazing results for his patients. Devang is also a strong believer in wrapping the excellent dental treatment with a very caring attitude which makes it a very pleasant journey for his patients. He holds very high dental standards and values and is very precise in his work.

I have been fortunate to have had the pleasure to shadow quite a few life-changing treatments that he provided to his patients. Devang is a great believer of the concept "If you can't explain it simply, you don't understand it well enough." He is very methodical in his approach and simplifies concepts and presents them in a clear and step wise format. Devang is a natural teacher and strongly believes in sharing his knowledge and skill set so he can make a bigger impact. He enjoys teaching and I greatly admire his passion and dedication to help other dentists. I am grateful for having Devang as my mentor. As you turn through the pages of this book the concepts of occlusion will become very clear and the application of these concepts in everyday dentistry will make routine dentistry very comfortable and smooth.

As John F. Kennedy has once said "we must find time to stop and thank those people who have made a difference in our lives". So, I would like to say "thank you" to Devang who has guided me throughout my career and I am sure this book will add great value to the readers. I hope Devang's teaching will be a life-changing moment for you in the same way it has been for me.

Dr Swetha Kantareddy

BDS

Acknowledgements

A number of people have played an important role in my life and without them I would not have been who I am, nor would I have written this book. So it is only fair that I say my thanks to the people who have helped me.

First of all, I would like to thank all members of my family and especially my mum for making me who I am, always believing in me and never questioning my ambition and for supporting me, even when it meant that I had to live on a different continent. I understand as a parent how painful this can be, so this book is for you, mum.

I would also like to thank my mentors who have helped me from the beginning of my dental career and pushed me to achieve great success and setting the standards so high from the beginning. Without them I would not have been in a position to write this book.

Last but in no way least, I would like to thank my wife and my son. For me family means everything and family always comes first. Yet I have spent countless weekends away on courses, studying and teaching, which meant away from my family, from the two people I love the most. Thank you for giving me that freedom to pursue my passion. Thank you, my son, for forgiving me for not spending time with you while you were very young.

Dr Devang Patel

P.S. I bribed my 7 year old son while writing this book by saying that if he gives me time to write this book then I will give him the opportunity to contribute to the book.

So here is what Ansh has to say,

"Thank you, Daddy, for giving me this opportunity to write in your book. I love you so much. You are an amazing dad. I am so proud of you and your achievements. You are an inspiration and your passion to help other dentists is amazing. Now that you have completed the book, let's play ☺"

Links to Further Materials

Your training goes beyond this book. Please use the links below to access the various additional resources that come free with this book.

They will be introduced throughout the book, however I have listed them below for your convenience.

Online Practical Guide to Full Mouth Reconstruction Book Course; use code **"fmrbook"** and the course will be free for you.

Full Mouth Reconstruction for GDPs Facebook Group:

Comprehensive Clinical Assessment E-Book:

If you are having any issues accessing any of the links by using the QR codes, then please make sure to contact me at https://drdevangpatel.com/contact/.

Feel free to connect with me on social media, I would love to hear from you and help you out further to be the most successful you can be in your career:

Facebook: Dr Devang Patel
Instagram: @dr_devangpatel
LinkedIn: Dr Devang Patel

You can also visit my website for more information and resources:

www.drdevangpatel.com.

Introduction

I have been practicing dentistry for around two decades and have treated hundreds of complex cases which required increasing Occlusal Vertical Dimension (OVD). I have been teaching the same subject for over a decade. In order to help General Dental Practitioners (GDPs), I have developed a pathway to full mouth reconstruction for GDPs. I help GDPs via an online course, a hands on course and if needed I can go to their practice to help them carry out their first case.

My experience has shown me that any general dentist regardless of their experience can carry out full mouth rehabilitation if they are dedicated and focused. I have taught dentists with less than 5 years of experience who are now doing full mouth reconstruction. I have also seen that you do not need to do any certificate courses or diplomas or MSc in order to do full mouth reconstruction. All you need is a structured approach and dedication towards learning and implementation. One of the most important aspects of learning is mentoring. I have been lucky enough to get mentored by some of the best mentors in the world and hence I was able to master many clinical skills such as full mouth reconstructions (restorative and implants), bone grafting procedures including autogenous bone grafting and sinus lifts, soft tissue grafting etc. rapidly and with great success. Hence, if you would like to learn full mouth reconstruction, then I urge you to find a mentor.

Although direct mentoring is irreplaceable, it is my sincere hope that this book will provide that valuable guide for those who are unable to gain direct mentoring but would like to start their journey with full mouth reconstruction.

I always advise dentists who are embarking on their journey to full mouth reconstruction to carry out direct adhesive restoration. The reason is that it is easy to manage and you can control occlusion very easily without relying too much on your technician. Once you have four or five direct cases under your belt you can start venturing into more complex cases. Of course, it is difficult to find cases where every single tooth is a direct restoration and hence you need to be prepared to do indirect restoration but the majority of restoration needs to be direct.

In order to carry out direct adhesive full mouth reconstruction predictably you need to understand the three fundamental steps which are involved in the process.

Step 1 is understanding occlusion and treatment planning. If you think about it, oral rehabilitation is nothing but a collection of single tooth restorations such as composite bondings, crowns, onlays or veneers which work harmoniously due to occlusion.

Once you have an understanding of occlusion and you have planned your case, you can start with ***step 2*** which is reconstruction of anterior teeth. These can be done using the direct, indirect or semi direct method. Sometimes you just need to carry out anterior reconstruction for the patient and using the DAHL technique, let the posterior teeth come into occlusion.

However, many patients do not fall under the criteria of DAHL technique and hence they will need posterior reconstruction which is ***step 3*** of the process. Posterior reconstruction can also be carried out using direct/indirect or semi direct methods.

I have written this book to be a practical guide for dentists who want implementable tips rather than theoretical research. Hence, I have not given references in any chapter, however, at the very end I have recommended books and some papers which I feel would help you further your knowledge.

I have also written this book to help general dental practitioners understand in detail the various practical steps involved in carrying out direct full mouth reconstruction.

This book is divided into three parts.

In Part One I will discuss occlusion and treatment planning, while in Part Two, I will look at anterior reconstruction. Part Three will seek to explain posterior reconstruction. They each contain the steps you can expect to follow while carrying out a full mouth reconstruction.

This process is aimed at beginners, teaching them practical points to help them complete direct build-ups. I believe the method taught here is the simplest and safest way to start doing full mouth reconstruction because if you make any errors, they will be easy to rectify.

I therefore believe it will provide a solid foundation for dentists who are confident in single tooth dentistry and are now ready to embark on treating more complex cases.

This book, unlike any other book, is LIVE. Yes, it is LIVE as you can follow the latest developments and techniques by signing up to the special course for all the dentists who have purchased this book where you will find numerous videos to go along with it. I will also share with you regular updates or any change of techniques as I develop new systems. Furthermore, communication is an important skill to have when you are doing any type of dentistry and it becomes even more important when you are doing full mouth reconstruction. Hence, as a gift from me to you,

I have also made my 'Communication in Dentistry' course available to you for free. You will get access to this course when you enroll into the book course.

You can access the free Online Practical Guide to FMR Book Course here:

https://drdevangpatel.com/courses/practical-guide-to-full-mouth-reconstruction/

When purchasing the book course, use coupon code 'fmrbook' and it will be free for you. The Communication Course is included there as well.

The Mindset of a Full Mouth Reconstruction Dentist

Before you start learning about or doing full mouth reconstruction, you need to understand the thinking behind it.

This may sound more mindset-oriented than skill-oriented but it is a vital part of the journey towards really understanding and believing that you can begin this important stage in your career - not least because numerous dentists have various self-limiting beliefs on this subject.

Let us look at some of the limiting beliefs of dentists I have come across in my teaching career.

"I'm not good enough"

For starters, many dentists have told me that they don't feel good enough or do not have enough experience. I have taught dentists who have over 20 years of experience and some who are barely two years into their careers, and what they have in common is that they all feel inadequate.

In my opinion it is not about experience - it is about exposure and attitude. Many times I hear such self-doubting thoughts from dentists who are clinically very good, and they don't realise that they just have a mental block.

This treatment can be done by anyone with a sound understanding of single tooth dentistry. That is why I have written a book designed to provide a clear pathway to success as well as theoretical knowledge. I am under no illusion that it is possible to start full mouth reconstruction by just reading a book or that it can replace invaluable experience you get while doing hands on courses and direct mentoring, but I am hoping to provide you with a step by step guide to help you understand the process.

"This isn't my specialism"

Another limiting belief is that you have to be a specialist. I am not one, despite having two masters' degrees. Sometimes different countries' attitudes towards specialisms will vary, but for the most part the days are long gone where you have to specialise to do this kind of treatment. You only need to learn the skills and put in hard work - then your dentistry will be world-class.

"It's too difficult to learn"

The third limiting belief is that it is very difficult to learn full mouth reconstruction. I have tried to address this by writing the steps in the book in such a simple way so as to make the principles straightforward and understandable.

"It's too expensive"

The fourth myth I often hear is "I need a lot of money to do the right courses". It's true that spending the money up front can feel daunting. Yet paying X amount for the courses which will return your investment within six months to a year, with some hard work and effort, is a very small investment considering the skills learned is for lifetime and the return is exponential over lifetime.

You just need to do one case to get your money back from paying for a hands-on course, and when a course is online, you sometimes only need to do less than half a case to be reimbursed.

In other words, the first case will make you break even, but the second, third, and fourth cases will bring in the profits. From an investment perspective, it's a no-brainer. This book will give you the confidence to start that journey.

"My boss won't support me"

The fifth major stumbling block I tend to hear from associate dentists is that "My boss will not invest in the right equipment or materials. Therefore, there's no point in doing the courses".

Again, this is a very limiting belief, as you can invest in the appropriate equipment and materials yourself. They will quickly pay for themselves. Don't let your boss limit your ambitions!

"What if I fail?"

The sixth major myth circulating around this subject is that the complicated nature of oral reconstruction will lead to low rates of success.

Everyone experiences "fear of failure", but it should never prevent you from learning anything new. And any mistakes are a chance to learn!

Again, this is the reason I have written this book, to demystify the process of full mouth reconstruction.

To learn more, a hands-on course, and possibly mentoring, may be necessary afterwards, which I offer for any UK-based dentists needing one-to-one help with full mouth reconstruction cases, providing an environment where it is safe for you to try things out. If you are not in the UK then I recommend you find someone local who can help you progress your journey or join me online.

You have all the steps in front of you, and the support you need – and just by reading this book you will have the theoretical knowledge you need to carry out your first case.

"My patients can't afford it"

It's worth finally mentioning that many dentists tell me they don't have patients who can pay for full mouth reconstruction in the area or system they work in.

I have worked in 15 different practices in the UK, from the richest parts of central London to some of the poorest parts of the countryside. I have seen no difference in case acceptance rates.

If anything, there is more of a need and desire for good quality dentistry in less affluent areas, as many patients are unlikely to have been to a dentist for some time and often feel desperate to make some changes due to their deteriorating oral health. Therefore, you will always have patients who will be willing to pay to improve their situation.

During my communication course, which you will have access to once you enroll into the online *Practical Guide to Full Mouth Reconstruction Book Course*, I will cover how to see patients for 15-minute checkups and use that time to communicate the full month reconstruction process effectively. More patients in need of treatment will then be able to access the right care.

For patients concerned with the cost, adhesive full mouth reconstruction is inexpensive by nature compared to conventional reconstruction, so it will be less likely to hurt the patient's pockets.

In my experience patients in the UK are under-treated rather than over-treated. Mild to moderate wear cases are often ignored or just result in patients being placed under monitoring. It is still essential to make sure you assess each patient properly before you decide what is best for them.

"Learn from the best"

If you're still skeptical, try seeing which dentists near to you have been doing this work, and learn from them.

Doing your research is important, as many dentists who do this kind of treatment are not vocal about it; therefore you will never know about them unless they go on Facebook, Instagram or Youtube to show off their cases. Figure out who is doing this and where, understand what each one is doing differently, and emulate any examples of best practice. If you would like to learn from the success stories of some of the dentists then listen to my podcast called '***The Ultimate Dentist Podcast***' which is available on Spotify, Apple Podcast, Google podcast and Stitcher.

If you would like to increase or improve your skill level, then you need to immediately reduce such limiting beliefs. Remember that if you are a general dental practitioner, you are in a great position to do full mouth reconstructions because you see plenty of patients.

The benefits of learning full mouth reconstruction

- **Holistic treatment planning**
  My favorite aspect of full mouth reconstruction is the ability to do holistic treatment planning. You are giving the patient a whole smile, not just improving one tooth or whitening or bonding one incisal edge. You are doing comprehensive dentistry and for most patients this will be life-changing.

- **Increased patient satisfaction and better aesthetic outcomes**
  Patients undergoing this treatment will almost always experience greater levels of satisfaction because the changes are so dramatic. You will also get predictable results because doing many restorations at once gives you a lot more control.

In turn this gives the patient a better aesthetic outcome compared to if you just conformed the treatment to the patient's existing occlusion.

- **Increased job satisfaction**
  You may love your job. Yet doing full mouth reconstruction is a completely different discipline because patients will also come to love your job. You see them many times, allowing you to build up a relationship and experience that great moment where you give someone their smile back, knowing they are your patient for life.

- **Increased earnings**
  You are going to earn more, and earning more will help you invest in your education. It's a virtuous circle.

Next steps: occlusion

You might now be saying to yourself "Okay, so how do I cross the bridge from being a dentist who restores single teeth to a dentist who does full mouth reconstruction?

Or you may ask the question "I'm already doing single-tooth dentistry and I'm very comfortable with it. I can do crowns, onlays and veneers, but how can I go further"?

There is a huge difference between doing 28 single crowns and a full mouth buildup; yet what makes the jump from one to the other possible is understanding occlusion.

In the following chapters we are going to discuss occlusion and the benefits of understanding it in more detail. You need to learn it first and foremost before you embark on full mouth reconstruction cases.

I hope by now you are convinced that learning full mouth reconstruction will be hugely rewarding, for yourself and for your patients.

If so, read on.

CHAPTER 1

Understanding Occlusion

1.1 The Importance of Occlusion in Oral Rehabilitation

In this section we are going to discuss the role of occlusion in full mouth reconstruction, focusing on why it is important.

You might think occlusion is irrelevant for anyone who isn't doing full mouth reconstruction cases. Therefore, let's first look at why you need to learn about occlusion.

Why bother learning about occlusion?

- **Replacing an old amalgam**
  Have you ever had to remove an old amalgam filling or restoration, replacing it with a lovely new composite restoration, but when you asked the patient to close his or her mouth, you found the occlusion was too high? You are then left with the frustrating task of grinding that composite out, leaving you with a really flat or faceted composite again.

- **Preparing a second molar for a crown**
  Similarly, have you ever had a case where you prepared a second molar, using a guide to make sure you left enough space for your final restoration but found that the crown is high and you are now grinding that crown down, so much so that it might be perforated or paper-thin in one or two points?

- **Treating patients who repeatedly break or chip restorations or teeth**
  Or maybe you have had a case where you treated a patient who repeatedly kept breaking one or more of the restorations?

- **Predictable comprehensive treatment to your patients**
  Perhaps you simply want to learn predictable dentistry, as well as dentistry which lasts?

If you are seeking an answer to any of these questions, you need to cover occlusion. This section of the book will help you do just that.

Let's look at the tooth in ***Figure 1a***. You can see there is a fractured cusp as well as faceting on the amalgam. It tells you that the tooth is a functional tooth and there was some kind of guidance coming from it.

It could be that the patient is bruxist or has some parafunctional habits, but what we don't know is whether there is an opposing tooth and the possibility of non-working side contact on that cusp. Yet you can see that the tooth was under a heavy occlusal load, otherwise there would not be faceting on the amalgam. It is the same for the tooth in ***Figure 1b***.

FIGURE 1a

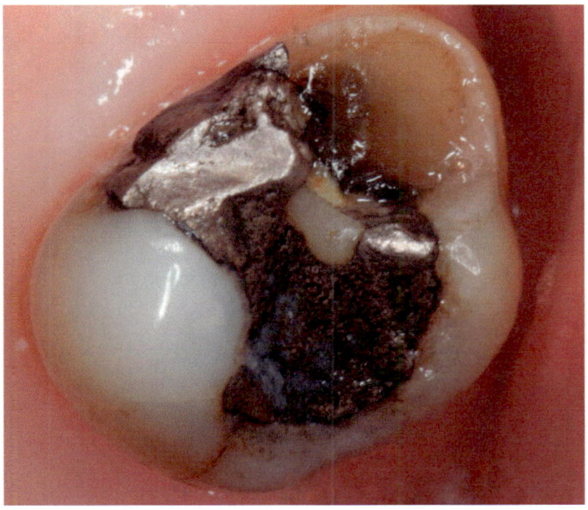

FIGURE 1b

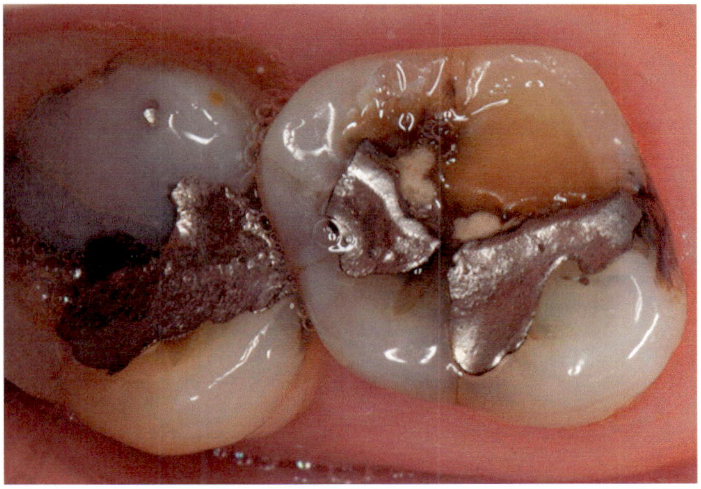

In ***Figure 2*** you can see that this second molar is split in half vertically and therefore needs to be extracted.

It's quite common to have cracks associated with amalgam, possibly to the point of fracturing (as was the case with the tooth in the previous picture). Yet occlusion could have been the culprit due to the huge faceting on the palatal cusp.

It's therefore important to find out what type of movements patients are making in order to create these types of occlusal faceting.

FIGURE 2

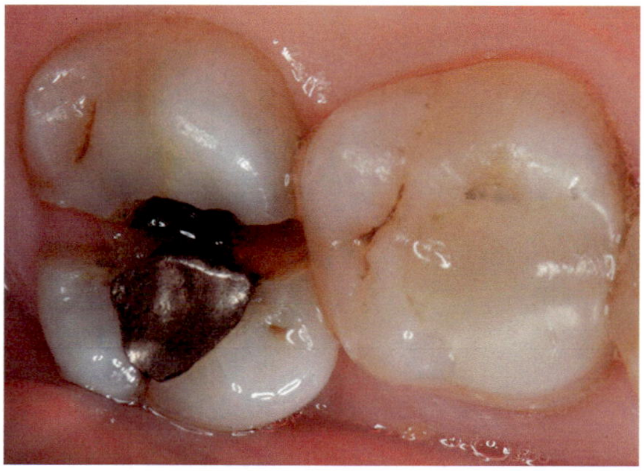

Figures 3a and ***3b*** show that the tooth was vertically fractured and we had to extract it.

FIGURE 3a

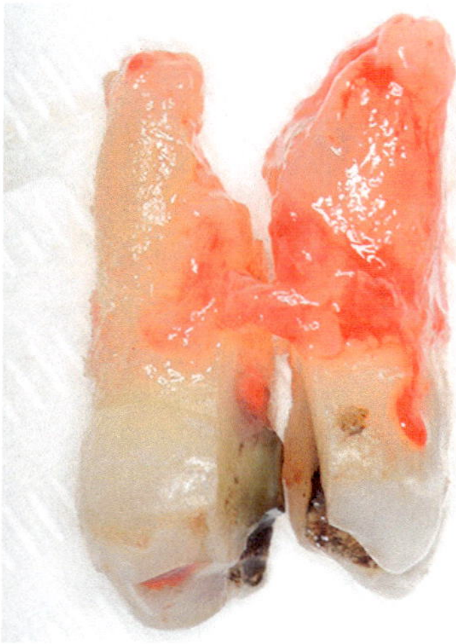

FIGURE 3b

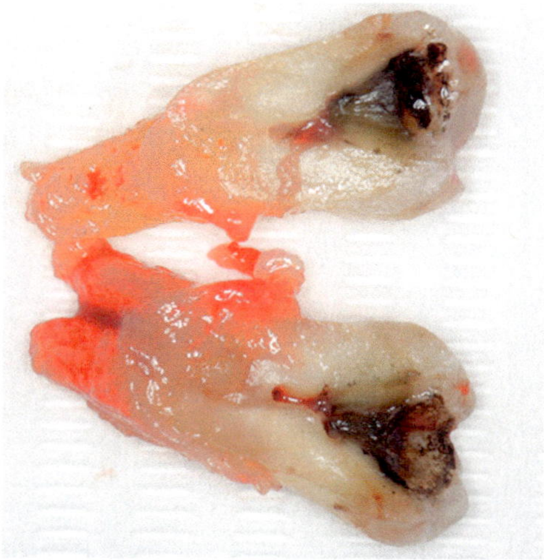

The example in ***Figure 4*** shows a vertical fracture within the functional cusp of the tooth.

We know that amalgam could be one of the causes; but understanding how to do an occlusal assessment is the key. It will show you whether the cusp had non-working side contact or working side contact, and whether it was grinding on the area and so might have caused the palatal cusp to break.

Therefore, you need to be able to figure out why this palatal cusp broke by doing an occlusal assessment, because when you're re-restoring the tooth then you need to make sure that you don't repeat the mistake that made it break in the first place.

FIGURE 4

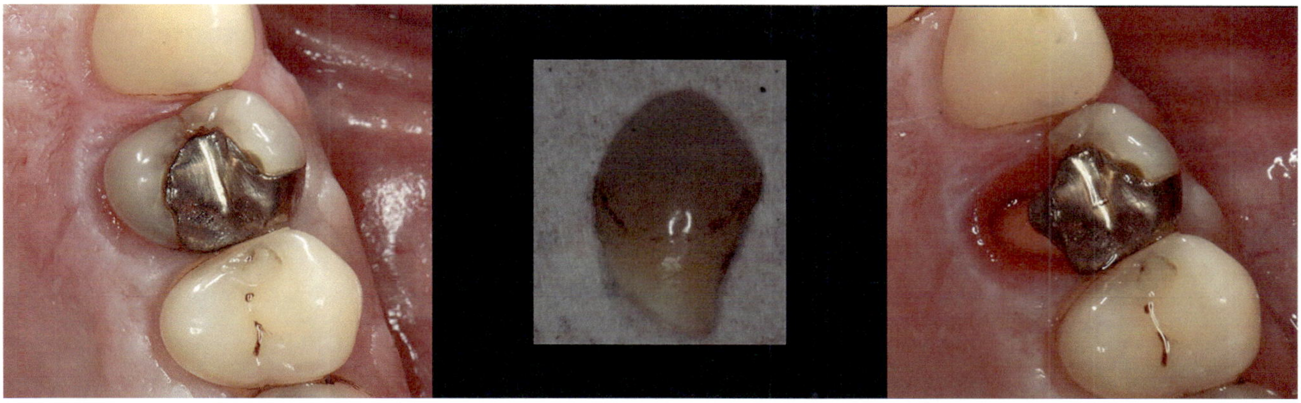

Why do teeth break?

- **Tensile strength – unfavorable load**

  One of the reasons teeth break is because of their tensile strength. Teeth get an unfavorable load placed on them because the edges are very sharp. Sharp edges lead to higher levels of tensile force, and tensile force will make things break.

  You want your teeth to experience compressive force as much as possible, and the restoration to experience both compressive and tensile forces.

  Of course, we cannot always avoid tensile forces, so it's advisable to have the cusps' tips be a bit flatter. If they're quite thin and sharp you will create lots of excessive tensile force.

  Another example of tensile strength gone wrong is when you have unsupported porcelain on a metal ceramic or zirconia crown with layered porcelain.

  When you have unsupported porcelain there is a higher risk that you will see porcelain fractures or chipping because the material has been subjected to tensile rather than compressive forces.

- **Fatigue – high risk among patients with strong masseters**

  Teeth can also break because of fatigue. Patients can experience cyclic fatigue on a tooth that has been exposed to non-working side contact. It's worth remembering this point, as we will explore it in more detail later on in the book.

- **Concentration of force – protruding lower incisors can be risky**
  Breakage due to an over-concentration of force is very common. In some cases you will see the lower anterior teeth are proclined and one anterior tooth will be protruding slightly above the occlusal plane.

  If you're doing an upper anterior restoration, it will fail if that tooth hits it, debonding any veneers a patient might have in the process.

  You may be wondering why you haven't encountered any of these issues, even if you have been doing dentistry for years. For most patients, their teeth will perform their function slightly apart, not really grinding except for when they swallow or reach the end of a chewing cycle.

  Contrary to what we used to believe, we know that when patients chew food right at the end of a cycle their teeth touch very gently and quickly, signaling to them to stop closing further and open their mouth to start chewing again.

  It's why many times when you do full mouth restorations, patients will complain about not being able to chew food properly because of the altered sensation involved when the teeth make premature contact. It's worth being mindful of this.

The differences between function and parafunction

Table 1:

Factor	Function	Parafunction
Duration of tooth contact per day	4-10 min	Up to 4 hours
Magnitude of applied force	20-40 lbs per sq. Inch	Up to 300 lbs per sq. Inch.
Direction of applied force	Vertical	Horizontal or Lateral
Level	Class III	Class I or II
Type of muscle contraction	Isotonic	Isometric (poor blood supply, build up of lactic acid resulting in cramps and spasms)
Proprioceptive Influence	Neuromuscular protective mechanism present	Neuromuscular protective mechanism absent
Mandibular closure position	ICP	Eccentric
Pathological Effect	None or at least minimal	Pathological changes, vary in different patients

For functioning patients, their teeth-to-teeth contact time is only four to ten minutes. For parafunctioning patients, teeth-to-teeth contact time could be up to four hours. The magnitude of that force is 20 to 30 lbs for normal functioning patient compared with 300 lbs for those that are parafunctioning.

The direction of force when patients are functioning is more vertical and compressive, whereas when patients are parafunctioning it is horizontal or lateral, which means exposing the teeth to greater levels of tensile force.

You can expect to perform a class 3 lever action when patients are functioning, whereas for patients who are parafunctioning it will be a class 2. A class 3 lever is less destructive than a class 2 lever due to the forces on the teeth.

Patients experience isotonic movement when functioning, whereas patients who are parafunctioning tend to experience isometric motion, the result of poor blood supply which leads to the muscles starting to ache. It becomes a continuing cycle.

When patients are parafunctioning, their neuromuscular system is absent as the body is either concentrating on something else or the patient is sleeping. Because of this, these patients can apply a bigger load to their teeth without knowing it.

The mandibular position is also different in this instance. A functioning patient will usually chew and close their mouth in a way that allows for maximum intercuspation, whereas with a parafunctioning patient their bite can go in any direction.

One way to figure this out is to line up any facetings - they are an amazing way to find out in which direction the grinding is happening. You therefore need to really look at the faceting in a patient's mouth to try and see if both jaws will meet together in that facet. If you get them to meet, you will know what kind of mandibular movement the patients are doing when they are grinding. This will help you understand whether the patient's chewing pattern is vertical or horizontal.

We know that Posselt [1952] told us that occlusion is one of the basic building bricks of dentistry. Yet this gives rise to two questions: why are we still struggling to understand occlusion? Why does it seem to be so perplexing?

Why is occlusion confusing?

- **It is not very well taught at the undergraduate level**
  One reason dentists have a mental block with occlusion is that it is not very well-taught in most undergraduate courses. Many universities don't have a separate subject called occlusion, teaching it within different subjects rather than giving it special attention.

  There are some exceptions, with a few universities having proper modules dedicated to it. However, this is still unusual.

- **There is too much information that seems difficult to relate to clinical practice**
  Even dentists can experience information overload. One dentist that I know has done four different courses on this subject yet is still unable to apply that information in her clinical practice because each teacher provided a different approach.

- **There are differing views**
  Opinions vary on how to treat full mouth reconstruction. Some experts advocate starting with posterior reconstruction first, while others advocate beginning with anterior reconstruction.

  Furthermore some would say that you need to restore cases in **Centric Relation (CR)**, while others would say there is no point in restoring patients in **Centric Relation (CR)** when you can restore cases in ICP. The possibilities are endless.

- **Lots of different terminologies to describe the same situation**
  Lots of different words exist to describe what is essentially the same thing. We will cover this more extensively in the chapter on terminologies, but for example CR, meaning centric relation, was known as CO two decades ago.

  However, we know now that they mean different things; CO refers to the first point of contact when patients are relaxed and CR is the name for the position the teeth adopt when they are apart and the jaw is in the most relaxed position.

  So, if someone first learned about occlusion in the 1990s, they might see CR or CO as the same thing. Hence, make sure you know your terminologies!

- **No scientific evidence**
  There is no scientific evidence suggesting that one way is superior over any of the others, such as whether you use a facebow or not or whether you apply canine guidance or a group function.

- **Conformative dentistry works most of the time**
  You need to really understand not just the science but also the art of occlusion. As we discussed, conformative dentistry works really well most of the time and hence you may be forgiven for not knowing occlusion when doing simple dentistry. However, if you do not know occlusion when doing full mouth reconstruction you may encounter serious problems.

- **A lot of practice is needed and cannot be learned by just reading books**
  If you decide to do a course on occlusion you will need to implement what you have learned in your practice and start trying things out on your patients. What's key here is practice, practice, practice.

  Oh, and don't forget to have someone next to you to check what you're doing!

Mistaken beliefs dentists have about occlusion and full mouth reconstruction

- **It's just for elites/specialists**
  Many dentists feel it's only for elite specialists. Yet as was mentioned before, nothing could be further from the truth.

- **It's just about canine guidance**
  Some dentists believe that all you need is canine guidance, building all the teeth and occlusion, and that's all there is to it. I fervently hope you will not agree with this point of view once you have read this book.

- **You only need to know occlusion for full mouth reconstruction**
  Again, this is a myth, as even if you're doing single-tooth dentistry you will need to know about occlusion.

  It's important to understand that a subject might seem confusing, but that doesn't mean it's complicated - which brings us on to the next point.

- **The subject is very complex**
  This subject is not very complex; many people think it is because of what surrounds it.

  The way you have to think about occlusion is that a patient needs to be able to close their teeth properly without having any discomfort and without having unnecessary forces concentrating on one or two teeth.

They should be able to chew properly without having any issues with a restoration. Therefore, all you need to check is the dynamic and static position of the teeth.

We only have 32 teeth in our mouths but dentistry is still a vast subject. Therefore, the key with occlusion is to start with simple first principles.

The benefits of learning about occlusion

- You will become better at **treatment planning** because you can plan full mouth reconstruction cases.
- You will be able to give patients a better **aesthetic result.**
- What's more, if occlusion is applied correctly then you will be able to give patients **predictable results**.
- In turn, your **productivity** will increase because you won't have to keep calling the patient back in again and again and again.
- Levels of **patient comfort** will increase because patients will be able to chew better.
- Even if they are grinding they can do so harmoniously, **decreasing levels of stress**.

Remember: learn the basics first and advance at your own pace from there.

My hope is that by the time you finish reading this book you will have a complete understanding of the steps involved in direct adhesive full mouth reconstruction.

1.2 Occlusal Terminologies

In this chapter we are going to discuss terminologies relating to occlusion, which is a vital part of understanding the process. It will also help you carry out full mouth reconstruction cases and communicate well with colleagues or mentors. Last but not least, it will assist you in getting the most out of any further reading on the subject you might do.

What is occlusion?

There are two aspects of Occlusion:

1: *the act or process of closure or of being closed or shut off (dynamic occlusion/articulation)*
2: *the static relationship between the incising or masticating surfaces of the maxillary or mandibular teeth or tooth analogues (static occlusion)*

You will find all the terminologies we are going to discuss in the glossary of prosthodontic terms (GPT), freely available on Google. Please make sure you get the most up-to-date version.

What does this mean for you?

This means that you need to consider both aspects of occlusion when you are planning or executing your dentistry.

For example, if you're doing a crown preparation, you need to check the reduction of your preparation in static occlusion when the teeth are closed, but you also need to remember to check the reduction when in dynamic occlusion.

Therefore, ask the patient to do an excursive movement, to ensure you will not incorporate any non-working side contact.

Connected – occlusion

Occlusion is not only about teeth: it involves gums, muscles, temporomandibular joints and neuromuscular systems (***Figure 5***). It's all interconnected, so if one system goes wrong it will have repercussions elsewhere. Hence, it is important to have an understanding of all the systems and their effects on overall occlusion. In this chapter, we are going to concentrate on terminologies related to occlusion.

FIGURE 5

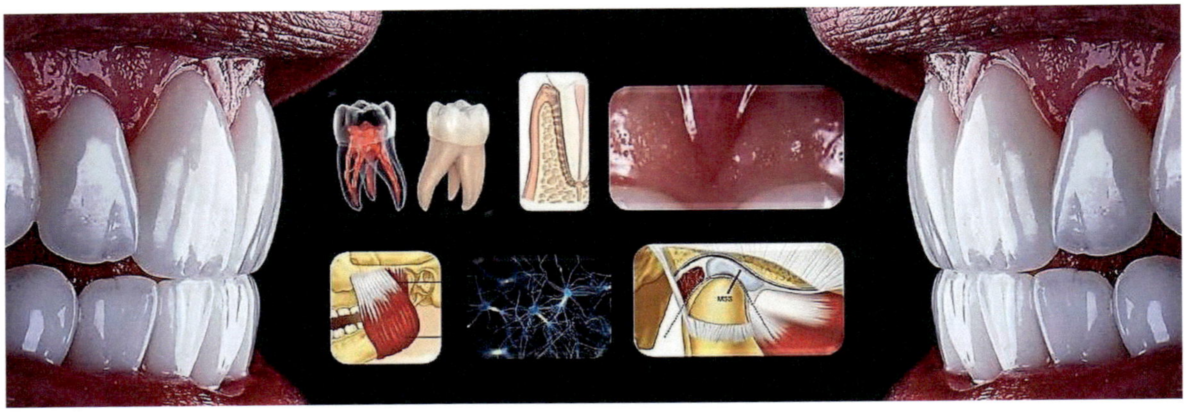

Terminologies

Let's look at some of the commonly used terminologies.

- **Centric relation (CR) or Retruded axis position (RAP)**

  Centric relation is defined as a maxillomandibular relationship, **independent of tooth contact**, in which the condyles articulate in the **anterior-superior position** against the posterior slopes of the articular eminences; in this position, the mandible is restricted to a **purely rotary movement**; from this unstrained, physiologic, maxillomandibular relationship, the patient can make vertical, lateral or protrusive movements; it is a clinically useful, **repeatable reference position.**

  It is an independent-to-tooth contact position, which means that when you are taking a record of the teeth they should be apart. It's very important to understand that the teeth have no influence on the position of centric relation.

- **Centric occlusion (CO) or Retruded contact position (RCP)**
  Centric occlusion is the occlusion of opposing teeth when the mandible is in centric relation, which may or may not coincide with the maximal intercuspal position.

  It also describes the relationship of the mandible to the maxilla, in which initial occlusal contact has occurred following closure during the centric relation (CR).

  This is a confusing term because it's not really an occlusion - it's the first point of contact, usually the cusp tip or the fossae or the occlusal area. From there on the jaw moves in what is usually a forward and upward direction and gets you maximum intercuspation (MI). The two jaws are nicely mish-mashed together.

- **Maximum Intercuspal Position (MI) or Intercuspal Position (ICP)**
  Maximum Intercuspal Position (MI) or Intercuspal Position (ICP) is the contact between the greatest number of opposing teeth while the mandible is stationary and in its most closed position.

Understanding centric relation

Centric relation is when:

- The **condyle-disc assembly** is the highest point possible – the anterior superior position. **The medial pole** of each condyle-disc assembly **is braced by bone. The inferior lateral pterygoid muscles** have released contraction and **are passive.**

  The inferior lateral pterygoid muscle has two bellies - the superior and the inferior. The inferior belly attaches to the condyle, the superior attaches to the articular disc, and needs to be passive and released of any contractions. Most TMJ problems happen because of the misfiring of the superior and inferior belly of lateral pterygoid muscle, which is why the lateral pterygoid is one of the most important muscles when it comes to understanding occlusion or TMJ problems.

- **The TMJ can accept firm compressive loading with no sign of tenderness or tension.** The other clinical implication is that when TMJ is in CR, it can accept firm pressure without any pain. This is relevant because you do not want to do full mouth reconstruction for patients who have tender TMJ under compression in CR. This can be checked by doing a 'load test'.

You need to address this issue first before you do any full mouth reconstructions to avoid post-treatment issues. Not all patients will come to you with easily recognizable symptoms and many of them might not even be aware of the problem.

How do you know you have a patient in CR when you are clinically assessing them?

Unfortunately, you will never know unless you are doing an MRI scan, which not every practice is set up for, and even then a slight movement when you're doing a scan can give you a false result.

Just make sure you've done your procedures properly - then you will have a predictable and repeatable position.

Why is centric relation so important?

- **Centric relation is a "tooth apart" position and has no influence on the teeth.**

  Because it's a "tooth apart" position and the teeth are not involved, it can be used as a guide for full mouth reconstruction cases where all teeth are being treated and hence ICP is not a reliable position as it will keep changing during the treatment.

- **Centric relation does not change over time and remains constant, except when changes in actual TMJ assembly occur. It is therefore repeatable.**

  Furthermore, CR does not change over time, so even if the teeth break or have restorations, the centric relation for that patient will not change unless there is an issue with TMJ and bone.

- **In extensive restorative cases where multiple occlusal surfaces are involved, the clinician cannot rely on ICP. Once the teeth are prepared it is very easy to lose habitual ICP as the patient develops new ICP, depending on the anatomy of the new restorations.**

  This is also important because being a 'teeth apart' position is a repeatable position. Once you open a patient's vertical dimension you lose all ICP contacts and that's why you need to rely on CR.

  When you're doing full mouth reconstructions and treating all the teeth, you can lose your guidance because you're now treating all the surfaces of the patient's mouth. You can still do a few quadrants or a few teeth at a time, but the whole purpose of doing full mouth reconstruction is to give you the space to restore a patient's teeth without damaging them.

❖ **This is a typical finding in natural dentitions and not a disease or diagnosis.**

It's natural, not patholcgical, and that's why we rely on CR.

CO to ICP slide

It is important to understand the concepts of CO and ICP slides. When a patient closes into their CR position and the first point of contact occurs between two teeth, that position is called CO (Centric Occlusion).

After that, in 90-95% of patients the jaw moves forwards and upwards to get maximum intercuspation because CO position is generally not the same as ICP.

❖ **CO only coincides with ICP in 5-10% of individuals.**

5-10% of patients see all their teeth mesh together rather than contacting CO first and then slide into ICP, which means that CO is in the same position as ICP. If this happens, you can use a leaf gauge or lucia jig to evaluate this position.

❖ **With everyone else, there is a slide between CO to habitual ICP. This is 1.25 ± 2.00 mm on average.**

In most patients, the slide is around 1-1.2mm horizontal and vertical, so patients will move forward for that distance. If you remove that slide then the patient's jaw won't be going forward - it will stay back and sometimes the patient may develop an anterior open bite as the mandible is no longer moving forward or sliding. This may be beneficial for you when you are treating a patient with tooth wear for full mouth reconstruction.

So, you need to find out where that first point of contact is and how much slide they have if you're planning to restore that tooth. This is one of the reasons why when you're preparing a second molar, and if that tooth was the one with CO, by doing tooth reduction you have also reduced the slide and hence the patient's TMJ will simply sit up more. This eventually closes the space and you lose the restorative space you created. It is very important to understand that!

- **The CO-ICP slide has horizontal and vertical components, and depending on the distance the slide can be called ''large vertical and small horizontal (Vh)'' or ''large horizontal and small vertical (Hv)''**

  The CO to ICP slide has two components: a horizontal component and a vertical one.

  In some patients the horizontal component is bigger which means the mandible goes further forwards before it goes upwards. And proportionately the forward movement is more than the upward movement. This is called 'Large horizontal and small vertical (Hv)'. In some patients it goes further upwards and then slightly horizontal which is called 'Large vertical and small horizontal (Vh). The majority of patients have Vh slides.

  Again, this is not one movement at a time. So it's going to be horizontal and vertical at the same time. If it's steep that means the patient has a large vertical and small horizontal, while if it's shallow that means the patient has more of a horizontal slide compared to a vertical one.

- **This slide is present in approximately 90% of the population and the average distance is 1mm-1.25mm.**

  The reason you need to know about this slide is because when you eliminate it in a patient with a large horizontal and a small vertical slide, then the patient is at high risk of developing an anterior open bite.

Figure 6 is an example of a large horizontal and small vertical case.
Figure 7 is a case where the patient has a large vertical and a small horizontal.

FIGURE 6

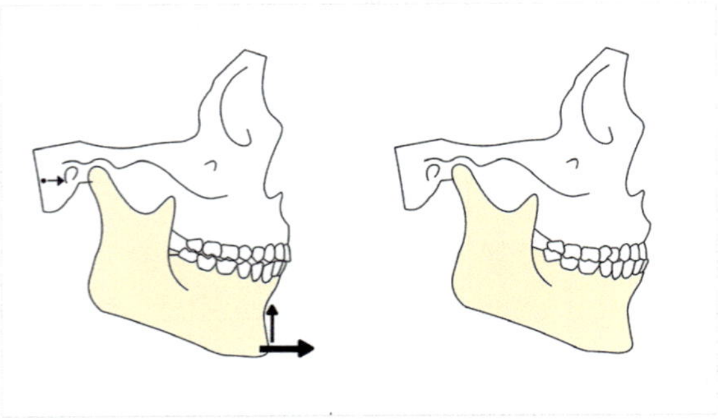

FIGURE 7

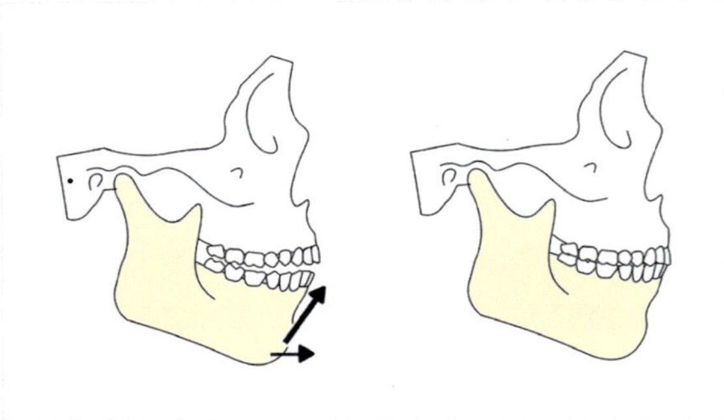

- **Alteration of the CO-ICP relationship is only undertaken when there are signs and symptoms to indicate that the patient cannot adapt to the magnitude or direction of the slide, or when reorganization offers a superior restorative result.**

  There are many theories around this. Lots of clinicians even suggest that if a patient's CO does not coincide with ICP, then you must correct this with an occlusal equilibration, as there are some studies suggesting that this is one of the reasons patients have TMD and occlusal issues.

  That said, there is no conclusive research on it, and my philosophy is that if a patient has natural dentition and no problems except this slide, then it's not pathological.

  However, if I'm restoring a patient's mouth doing full mouth reconstruction and I don't want to incorporate a slide, I'll make sure that I have created an occlusion where the CO is the same as the ICP.

  In short, a patient closing from CR straight to ICP is one way to overcome this issue.

- **Occlusal splint therapy to determine the likely outcome of such alterations is a wise precaution before proceeding, and is imperative if a patient is in pain.**

  If you find a patient who has pain in the TMJ or the muscles, then the best thing you can do is provide the patient with an occlusal splint such as a Michigan splint.

  Some terminologies you need to be aware of are listed below.

Working side contact

Working side contact means if patients move their jaw on their left the left side contacts become working side contacts, including whatever teeth are touching on the left side.

Non-working side contact

Non-working side contact occurs when patients move their jaw on the left and teeth that are touching on the right-hand side. They become non-working side contacts. Many times they have been described as occlusal interference.

However, I would personally not consider this as an interference, if a patient has natural dentition but experiences non-working side contact. In this case, it's best to just leave them alone.

Yet if you are restoring a tooth, you want to make sure that you don't incorporate non-working side contacts, because the forces are much higher on that tooth and they may break your restoration.

Condylar inclination

It's not really an inclination of condyles, but a fossa inclination and the angle at which condyle travels downwards. It is usually roughly 30 to 35 degrees. That's why on our articulator we keep the settings to 25 degrees, as by keeping the inclination shallow we will avoid interferences in the mouth when we use the articulator to form any restorations.

Curve of Spee

Another term you need to understand is the **Curve of Spee** (***Figure 8***), which happens if you simply draw a line between the cusp tip of the canine and join the buccal cusps of all the teeth till the last molar**.**

The relevance of this is if you have a flatter Curve of Spee, which I would recommend when you're doing a full mouth reconstruction, you can get away with a nice shallow anterior guidance. If you have a steep Curve of Spee then you will need a steeper anterior guidance, which may restrict the envelope of function and cause problems when patients are closing and opening and parafunctioning.

FIGURE 8

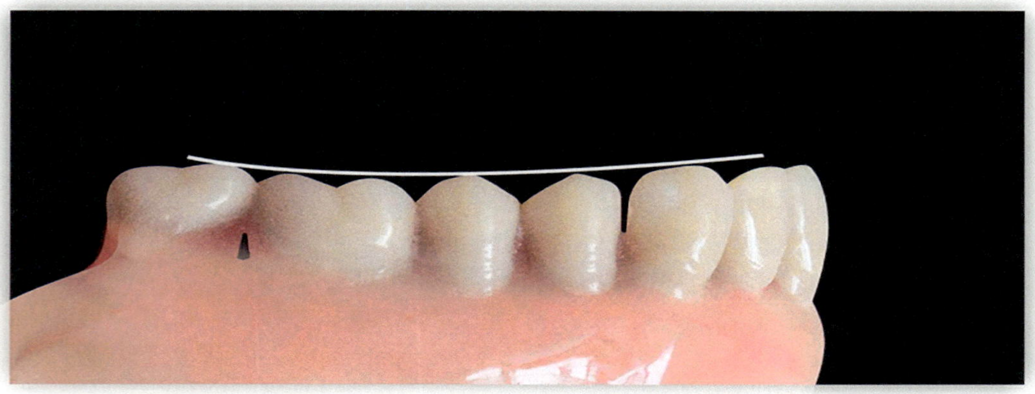

Curve of Wilson

The **Curve of Wilson** is a mediolateral cusp tip to cusp tip curve which helps us in chewing our food. Because the lower teeth are lingually inclined, it helps the buccinator muscle chew food in a nice position.

As a result, in the **Curve of Wilson** the circular motion is very important.

Anterior guidance

Many people confuse Anterior Guidance with protrusive guidance. Protrusive guidance is when you use your anterior teeth to make protrusive movements of the mandible.

When patients move their jaw forward that's called protrusive guidance. Anterior guidance is anything related to your teeth (including protrusive and lateral guidance), while posterior guidance is anything which is related to your TMJ assembly, including the joint and your muscles and the mandible, so you don't have any control over it.

Therefore, you only have control of your anterior guidance, which is teeth or tooth-related guidance.

Types of occlusion by disclusion

There are various different discussions. Let's look at them individually below.

- **Bilateral balanced occlusion**
  The bilateral balanced occlusion is mainly used in dentures so that when you give patients full dentures, you are trying to give guidance or occlusion. If a patient moves their jaw on the right side, the right and left side teeth will touch simultaneously. It's called balanced occlusion because everything is in contact at the same time.

- **Unilateral balanced occlusion** achieved via group function
  The unilateral balanced occlusion is when patients move their jaw to one side then all the teeth on that side are in contact but there is a disclusion on the other side. In an ideal unilateral balanced occlusion all teeth are used for guidance including molars, however generally when we are trying to achieve group function we would like to avoid using molars for lateral guidance.

- **Disclusion** achieved via canine guidance
  This is a process where only the canine is in contact while guiding on the same side and complete disclusion on the other side.

Types of discussions

- **Group function: During entire lateral movements the buccal cusp of the posterior teeth will be in contact. A distinction can be made between partial and complete group function depending on how many teeth are in contact.**

  The unilateral balanced occlusion is also called group function. Group function is simply when multiple teeth are in contact.

  Let's say when patients move their jaw on the right side all the teeth on the right side from the canine onwards are in contact. If more than one tooth is in contact but not all of them, then that is called partial group function.

  Full group function means all the teeth are in contact, but we usually aim for partial group function because closer we get to TMJ and muscles of mastication, lateral forces applied on the teeth gets heavier and hence can be detrimental to molars.

  Hence, it's best to try and limit things to premolars and canines, but if you have to include a molar then just use the mesiobuccal cusp of the first molar.

- **Canine guidance: During the entire lateral movement of the mandible there is no contact between the posterior teeth on either side. The canine on the working side will be the only tooth in contact during this movement.**

  Canine guidance and partial group function are the most frequently-used schemes. For sake of ease, from now on when I describe group function, I mean partial group function.

Group function

Group function and canine guidance are both equally important schemes and they have their own uses. Many dentists, including me, have preference on canine guidance but we must understand the scenarios when group function would be necessary.

Advantages of group function

- Group function allows a distribution of stress. This is the biggest advantage because you're not putting all the force on one tooth, allowing you to distribute the stress very nicely.
- It's conducive to reducing occlusal wear because you are reducing the stress on one single tooth.

Disadvantages of group function

- It is technically demanding and may not be successful without intraoral adjustment.
- That's why if you're doing an indirect restoration it becomes even more challenging because you really don't want to adjust any restoration too much; yet in order to get an ideal occlusion, you may have to adjust your indirect respiration.
- Therefore, it's important to try and use canine guidance whenever possible but understand how group function works, as there are multiple scenarios where you will want to reduce the stress and spread your guidance amongst the other teeth.

Indications of using group function:

- A class 1 occlusion with extreme overjet.
- A class 3 occlusion with all lower anterior teeth outside of the upper anterior teeth.
- Some end-to-end bites.
- An anterior open bite.
- When the canine is very weak and not suitable to take the load for a periodontal or restorative reason or if it's an implant restoration.

One scenario is when patients have class 1 overjet, where the canine is not in contact, or a class 3 when some of the end-to-end bite when a canine has got a very small surface means it's not big enough for you to create entire guidance on it.

This is why you may want to spread the guidance over both canines and premolars. If the canine is weak or an implant, then that is another reason to use group function.

Canine guidance

Why canine?

- Canines have a **favorable crown to root ratio.**

- Long roots mean more PDL ligaments, and because of that the tooth can have **more proprioception.**
- The **palatal surface** of the canine is ideal to create lateral guidance which is nice and shallow, and you can make it as deep as you want because it's a single surface.
- It's so **easy to manage mechanically.** It's in a favorable position because it's furthest from the muscles and so the load which the muscle can apply to that tooth is less.

Why canine guidance?

- Decrease in temporalis and masseter muscle activity with canine guidance rather than group function.
- During lateral movement, occlusal forces are more evenly distributed by canine guidance.
- Canine guidance reduces muscle activity during parafunction.
- Canine guidance is easy to deal with.

With regards to canine guidance, we know that it reduces the muscle activity during lateral movements and helps you in reducing this issue when patients are parafunctioning. But the reason I use it is because it's easy to manage.

Protrusive guidance

Protrusive guidance is usually provided by upper centrals and laterals, sometimes involving canines. If your centrals and laterals are missing you can use a canine to produce lateral guidance and protrusive guidance at the same time.

If canines and incisors are missing, then you can use the mesial slope of the premolar to give protrusive guidance. Ideally in most cases the front teeth will be present. Using them as protrusive guidance will make your life easier.

Four types of occlusal schemes to consider:

- Use of all central and lateral incisors and canines.
- Use of all central and lateral incisors.
- Use of canines alone.
- Use of mesial slope of premolars.

Factors deciding types of guidance

- Vertical and horizontal overlap of the anterior teeth as well as shape and axial alignment.
- Condition of the tooth/teeth.
- Ease of use.

You need to decide which guidance to choose when doing full mouth reconstruction. I use canine guidance when I can, but when I cannot use canine guidance then I will use group function.

A major reason for this is that canine guidance is very easy to manage and implement and you get more predictable results, whereas if you're going for the group function technique, making restorations will be a bit trickier, especially when you're doing an indirect restoration.

So canine guidance is generally easier. However, if the canine is an implant or is quite heavily restored or has a post and core crown or is not in occlusion because of an open bite or indeed, if there is no canine, you will need to rely on group function.

'Ideal' occlusion

So what are we really aiming for with full mouth reconstruction? The end goal is to have the teeth working and protecting each other when they are in contact.

When patients are doing excursive movements, we know that the posterior teeth will be under a lot of strain. During lateral movement you don't want too much force on the posterior teeth.

That's when anterior teeth take over and disclude posterior teeth immediately, which means there is no lateral force on posterior teeth. We know the anterior teeth are not that strong in the face of heavy compressive forces or vertical forces, which is why the posterior teeth take the vertical load.

Hence, when patients close their mouths gently, the posterior teeth are in heavier contact with each other than the anterior teeth. Anterior teeth have very light contact with one another when patients close in ICP, the result of the posterior teeth protecting the anterior teeth.

1.3 Comprehensive Occlusal Examination

In this chapter we are going to discuss the process of occlusal examination.

Whenever you are carrying out an occlusal examination on a patient, you are looking for signs and symptoms of parafunction, as this will be one of the main issues patients will come to you with when you're doing a full mouth reconstruction.

Signs and symptoms of parafunction

- TMJ
  You will find with TMJ that patients **may have pain or limited movement** of TMJ.

- Muscles
  Patients may come in experiencing **pain or myospasm within their muscles**, stopping them from opening their jaw properly.

- Teeth
  With regards to the teeth, the patient may have **wear faceting, fracturing of the teeth, drifting of the teeth or pain or hypersensitivity within the teeth.**

- Restorations
  They may have **wear or fracture or decementation** of their restoration.

You need to understand that when doing an examination, you will not find all these symptoms in one patient. You might have one or two symptoms. Then you need to diagnose and find out whether these symptoms are related to parafunction or something else.

This is where your occlusal assessment will be invaluable.

If a patient has all the symptoms, especially TMJ and muscle-related symptoms, you should not start with full mouth reconstruction. Instead you should make sure you reduce or remove those issues before you start with full mouth reconstruction.

You may stabilise those fractured teeth and any restorations, but before giving them any definitive treatment you need to make sure you address the TMJ and muscle issues.

Warning signs

What are the warning signs when a patient sees you for an assessment? How easily can you predict whether this patient has parafunctional habits and will be harder to treat?

- One thing you will see is that if you ask a patient to close their teeth together, they may not be able to close or even find a position where they can close comfortably.

Of course, there are patients that will move their jaw everywhere when they close; but I'm talking about patients who genuinely cannot close their teeth properly in one go because their muscles are very stiff and they cannot remember the right location.

- You will see that these patients will have multiple broken and worn-down teeth.
- TMJ or muscle pain.

These are the warning signs. We know that a patient who has parafunctional habits will be more difficult to treat or undertake full mouth reconstruction than a patient who just comes in with erosive wear.

What does the examination entail?

An **occlusal examination protocol** should include the following:

- A **TMJ assessment** for clicking, crepitus or pain.
- An assessment of the **muscles of mastication** such as the temporalis, masseter, medial pterygoid, lateral pterygoid and other extraordinary muscles in order to assess tenderness.
- An assessment of all the teeth as part of a full examination. This won't be our focus here, but it's still vital.

Occlusal examination:

- When you start doing an occlusal examination, you're going to assess a patient's **skeletal pattern.**
- You will discern whether they have a class 1, 2 or 3 occlusion.
- You're going to assess the **patient's overbite or jet.**
- **Assessing CO:** Check the first point of contact by using a leaf gauge, a very workable tool that I have demonstrated how to use in the online course called *Practical Guide to Full Mouth Reconstruction Book Course* which is free for the reader of this book.
- **Assessing ICP:** You are going to check the ICP to see if it is stable or unstable. If the patient cannot close their teeth properly and cannot 'find their bite' then it is unstable.
- You will see a **slide between CO to ICP.** If you don't have a leaf gauge you can assess by Bimanual Manipulation, noting whether the slide is a large vertical, small horizontal, small vertical or large horizontal, as we discussed in a previous lesson.
- Next you're going to assess the **shimstock holds of each individual pair of teeth**. Sometimes one tooth may contact two teeth on the opposing arch, which is noteworthy as it will help you assess your mounted models later on.

Assessing guidance/potential interferences:

Assessing lateral guidance

- You're going to assess the **Right Lateral Guidance** when the patient moves their jaw on the right side, you need to assess the teeth that are making contact on the right side (which are working side contacts) and the teeth contacting on the left side (which are non-working side contacts).
- You're going to repeat the same for the **Left Lateral Guidance**, making sure you check the teeth on the left side and then the teeth on the right side.

Assessing protrusive guidance

- This is the point where many dentists forget to check the protrusive guidance or check any interferences from the posterior teeth.

Therefore, when the patient moves their jaw forward, you should check the anterior teeth.

What you also need to do is put an articulating paper on the posterior teeth and see if any are in contact when the patient's jaw protrudes. That's how you assess protrusive guidance.

I hope this brief summary was informative.

1.4 Different Types of Occlusal Splints and Their Uses

In this chapter we are going to discuss occlusal splints and their uses.

Yet before we move onto this, let's remind ourselves of the differences between function and parafunction we discussed earlier in this chapter, as this is one of the main reasons along with TMJ and muscle issues, we provide occlusal splints for our patients.

What is an occlusal splint?

- An occlusal splint is any removable artificial occlusal surface affecting the relationship of the mandible to the maxillae, used for diagnosis or therapy.
- Possible uses for this device may include, but are not limited to, occlusal stabilization for treatment of temporomandibular disorders; diagnostic aid prior to extensive intervention; occlusal equilibration; and prevention of wear of the dentition or damage to brittle restorative materials such as dental porcelain.
- Hence, the splint is not only used for preventative reasons but it can be used for diagnosis and treatment purposes.

Effects of occlusal splints

Let's look at some of the effects of these splints, shown by the results of different studies.

- One effect is reduced EMG activity in nocturnal bruxism patients when they're using a splint due to relaxation of the muscles.
- We know from studies that patients with no dysfunctional activities can reproduce pantographic tracings, whereas patients with dysfunctional activities cannot reproduce pantographic tracings.

- However, studies have shown that if you give those dysfunctional patients splints such as Michigan splint, then many of them will be able to reproduce pantographic tracings, suggesting that their muscles are more relaxed.

Of course, these studies should still be subject to critical assessment because we know that not all EMG studies are fully accurate, due to various issues related to validity of the studies. But overall benefits of splints are proven in various studies.

However, we know from experience that occlusal appliances work in most scenarios. Therefore, let's look in more detail at the varied roles played by occlusal splints.

The role of occlusal splints

Splints serve three main purposes: diagnostic, preventative and for use in treatments.

Occlusal splints - diagnostic purpose

- **A splint helps to relax and deprogramme muscles of mastication in order to record the true CR when you want to mount your models accurately.**
  If patients have dysfunctional muscles and you cannot relax them using a lucia jig or a leaf gauge, then you may use a Michigan splint or similar long to medium term deprogrammer so that you can take true CR positions before you mount models - and maybe potentially do a full mouth reconstruction for that patient.

- **A splint is also helpful for assessing and trying out a proposed occlusal scheme at increased OVD.**
  When you're making a Michigan splint you can use a lucia jig or leaf gauge at a certain vertical level, which helps you in mounting models at certain OVD which you may decide according to need for the restorative space.

  If you use a Michigan splint in that restorative space, then that can help the patient get used to it. If the patient doesn't get used to that increased OVD, then that tells you that you have gone beyond the patient's adaptive capabilities.

  As a result, this patient may not be the ideal candidate for you to do full mouth reconstruction at that OVD as they cannot tolerate raising of OVD.

- **A Michigan splint can help you in assessing a patient's compliance.**
  If a patient cannot wear this splint before treatment, then you know that they may not be able to wear it post-treatment, leaving your restoration vulnerable to fracture and breakage.

- **The wearing down of a splint may suggest a heavy parafunctional habit.**
  If the splint is wearing down very rapidly then you know that there is a high chance that your restorations will also wear down, chip or fracture if the patient does not wear a protective occlusal splint during the night or while they are parafunctioning.

- **It helps you in the pre-restorative stabilisation of the TMJ, muscles and teeth.**
  By giving the patient a splint, you're providing them with relaxation of the muscles, an important process of stabilisation that happens before the treatment.

Occlusal splints – preventative purpose

- **Splints prevent further wear or tooth surface loss due to parafunctional habits.**
  Yet it is very important that you understand that it only *helps* against such habits.

  Dentists and patients are under the illusion that if you provide the patient with an occlusal splint then it will stop the progress of wear.

  Unfortunately that's not the case, as if a patient has worn down their teeth and the dentine is exposed, that dentine will continue wearing down within a normal function as well as during parafunction. Splint will only prevent wear during the duration of use of the splint.

  Even if patients stop parafunctioning, that dentine will continue wearing down, which is why those patients will need full mouth reconstruction or restoration to cover exposed dentine.

  It is necessary to make patients understand that if they don't want full mouth reconstruction, just giving them an occlusal appliance will not stop the ongoing wear because the dentine is exposed and will wear away much more quickly than enamel.

- **Protection of restorations.**
  When we do full mouth reconstructions, we need to give patients some sort of occlusal appliance to protect their new restorations.

Occlusal splints – treatment purpose

- **It helps with the management of TMD where occlusion is the main factor**

If occlusion is one of the main factors causing TMD and if you give a patient a Michigan splint or similar splint, then that should help in reducing the symptoms.

- **Stress-related pain symptoms, derived from hyper muscle activity**, are also reduced by giving the patient a splint.

- A splint can further reduce the effect of **trauma from occlusion and the mobility of the teeth.**
  It can help if a patient has dental **pain associated with occlusion.**

- A splint can similarly help in the **temporary removal of occlusal interference.** Although it's not a permanent solution, when a patient wears a Michigan splint you can eliminate interferences and study the outcome.

Types of splints

There are two different types of splints: directive splints versus permissive splints.

- A **directive splint** will help the patient guide that jaw in a particular direction, not allowing them to close in a different direction.
- By contrast a **permissive splint** allows the patient to move their jaw in all different directions, guiding them without restricting them.

Different types of splints:

1) Soft full coverage
2) Hard full coverage splint
   - Flat plane
   - Michigan/Tanner splint
3) Anterior repositioning appliance/Mandibular advancement splint
4) An Anterior Midpoint Stop Appliance (AMPSA) = NTI-tss (Nociceptive Trigeminal Inhibition - tension suppression system)
5) Mandibular Orthotic Repositioning Appliances (MORA) – directive splint
6) Posterior bite plane
7) Pivoting splint
8) 'B' splint
9) Hydrostatic splint

Let's look at them individually:

1) Soft full coverage splint

The soft full coverage splint (***Figure 9***) is one of the most commonly-used splints in general dentistry because it's easy to make a single impression and it protects the teeth from parafunctional habits. So if your aim is simply to protect a patient's teeth, then it will do the job.

FIGURE 9

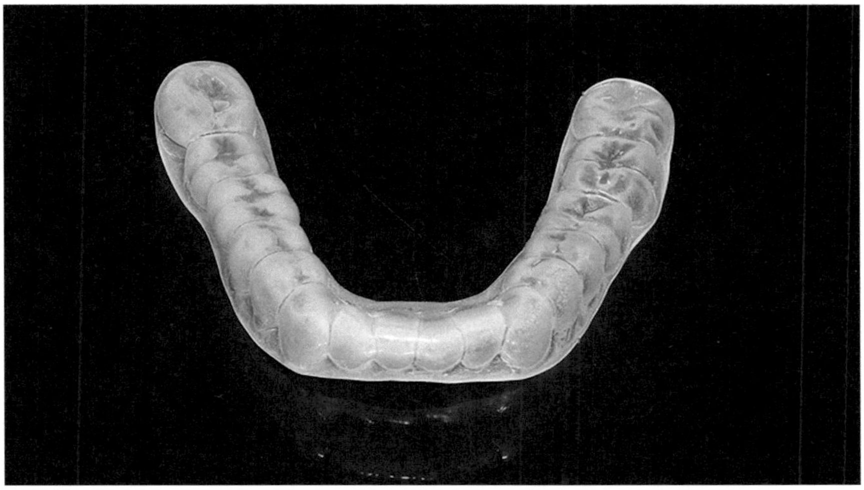

However, we also know from studies that if you give patients this kind of splint, it will act like chewing gum, which means a patient will grind the teeth more and more, damaging the splint and wearing it down. In other words, you may start a parafunctional habit by giving them this splint.

Having said that, if the patient doesn't have any TMJ problems and if you just want to protect any restorations for a short period of time, then these types of splints are helpful.

2) Hard full coverage splint

- **Flat plane**
- **Michigan/Tanner splint**

Flat surface splints are useful in giving some protection, however, the Michigan splint (***Figure 10***) or the Tanner appliance will be more useful for diagnostic, treatment purposes or preventative purposes.

FIGURE 10

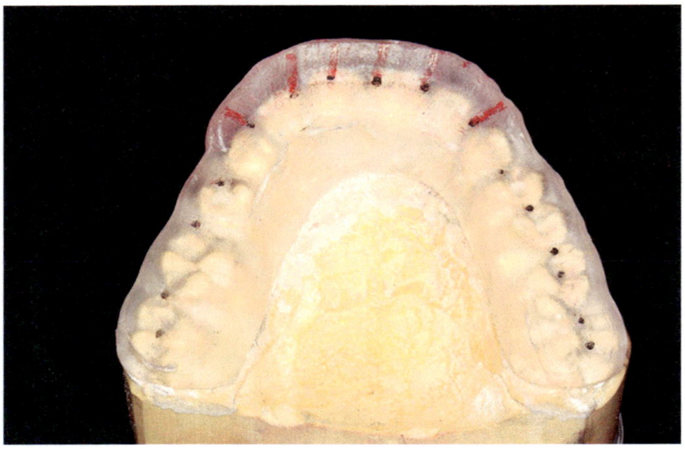

They create an idealised occlusion in a reversible manner, which means you can test your full mouth reconstruction case or occlusal scheme into that splint before you even start the treatment.

Furthermore, they guide condyles in CR, which are the most stable position in a musculoskeletal sense, and therefore help in reducing any issues with TMJs.

In turn, this reduces trauma from occlusion by distributing the load, which in turn reduces muscle pain due to the decrease in loading and muscle activity, and so temporarily reduces or eliminates interferences.

This is my choice of splint when it comes to full mouth reconstruction and hence, we will concentrate on the fabrication and use of this splint in this book.

3) Anterior repositioning appliance /mandibular advancement splint – directive splint

A Michigan splint (or soft splint) is a permissive splint which allows the patient to move their jaw in any direction, whereas with this splint the patient can only close in one direction. It is useful when patients have problems with clicking or TMJ issues with reduction of the capsule - even though it's often only helpful in the short-term.

4) An Anterior Midpoint Stop Appliance (AMPSA) / NTI-tss (Nociceptive Trigeminal Inhibition - tension suppression system)

It is like a Lucia jig, and you can rely on it as a very good tool for short-term use.

However, it comes with the risk of a patient inhaling or swallowing it during the night. Although it is rare, it can happen if the splint is loose.

If they use it for the long term, there is a risk that they will experience an intrusion of the anterior teeth or extrusion of the posterior teeth, developing an anterior open bite. To avoid this, advise the patient to use it for night time only.

That said, it does remove occlusal interferences, allowing freedom for the full seating of condyles and encouraging the release of lateral pterygoid muscles. So it can help a situation, but it is not fit for long-term use.

To avoid the issue of supraeruption, you can incorporate this type of appliance into a full coverage appliance where it simply covers the rest of the teeth without providing any contact with the opposing teeth, simultaneously preventing the risk of inhaling the appliance.

5) Mandibular orthotic repositioning appliances (MORA) – directive splint

This type of splint directs the lower jaw the patient can only close in one direction. Again, it is used to reduce the load on the TMJ and give the temporary mandibular joint and the capsule a little bit of relaxation.

6) Posterior bite plane

It is just a flat plane on the posterior occlusal surfaces, only leaving anterior teeth uncovered and raising the bite on a flat, hard occlusal surface. Many studies claim that it improves sports performance; however, this is not really proven as no robust analysis has been done in this area.

7) Pivoting splint

The pivoting splint is a splint where you have just one point of contact on either side and then the mandible can pivot again, reducing the load (or intracapsular load) on the TMJ for patients with TMJ problems.

8) 'B' splint or 'Dual B Splint'

B Splint is simply an Ess x retainer with an anterior ramp. It is a simpler solution to Michigan splint. And arguably more tolerable to patients.

If you want to give the patient a splint but you are worried about orthodontic retention, then the Dual B Splint is a good splint to use because it's a dual arch. You can give a patient a lower retainer and an upper splint will fit very well into that, acting as a deprogrammer and protector for your restorations.

9) **Hydrostatic splint**

The hydrostatic splint is used as a water-filled chamber for the posterior teeth, so when a patient closes their jaw the water will adjust and accommodate to the patient's bite. However, this kind of splint is almost obsolete and rarely used.

After looking at these different types of splint, it's very easy to get confused as to which splint should be used and when. A good guiding principle is that a Michigan splint or tanner appliance is still one of the most widely-used appliances by clinicians who carry out full mouth reconstructions.

Commonly used cheap substitutes, such as soft splints or bite guards, are only useful in the short-term for the immediate relief of acute pain, and cannot be used in the long term due to the issues discussed previously. They also cannot be used for diagnostic or treatment planning purposes.

How do you choose which splint to use?

- First and foremost**, diagnosis is key.** You need to make sure you've done the occlusal assessment to make sure you know what the patient's main problem is.

- As our main concentration for this book is full mouth reconstruction, the decision is easy. I use Michigan splint for almost everything, including pre treatment diagnostic use and post treatment preventative use. I use Dual arch B splint after completion of full mouth reconstruction for patients who need orthodontic retention.

- **If a patient has a TMJ disc displacement without reduction, you can give them a Michigan splint.**
  When patients have disc displacement without reduction, the patient cannot open completely because their disc has dislocated forwards and it cannot go back into its position.

  In these cases you can refer a patient to an oral surgeon or maxillofacial surgeon and see if they can do the required treatment; however, it is not the most predictable way to deal with this situation.

If you have referred a patient for surgery and the patient doesn't want surgery, then a Michigan splint helps with relieving the pain, as the ligament will stretch and the patient can regain some sort of normal regime of mouth-opening.

- **However, if the patient has a TMJ disc displacement with a reduction and clicking, then you can use the anterior repositioning appliance for three to four weeks to see if the symptoms reduce, followed by a Michigan splint.**
  If the symptoms don't decrease, you can increase the timing of that splint, but try to avoid giving more splint time than necessary.

You may not be able to completely reduce the clicking, but as long as the pain and the symptoms are gone you can go back to the Michigan splint for long-term usage.

As discussed, Michigan splint is my go to splint when it comes to doing full mouth reconstruction. So let's look at this splint more in detail in the next chapter.

1.5 Michigan Splint - Steps

In this chapter we are going to discuss the various steps involved in fabricating a splint.

As I discussed in the previous chapter the Michigan splint is one of the best types of splint for frequent use and certainly has advantages when it comes to full mouth reconstruction.

Michigan splint – things to consider

- **Assessment**

  Dentition is stable and free of caries, broken restorations and periodontitis

  You must make sure you have done a thorough assessment before giving this device to a patient. This should involve assessing a patient's dentition to make sure they don't have any cavities.

  If the patient has any broken restorations, then restore the teeth first. If a patient has periodontitis, make sure the periodontitis is under control before you give them a Michigan splint.

  A decision needs to be made about whether the splint will be used for diagnostic, preventative or treatment purposes.

  Make sure the patient understands the instructions for use before the procedure starts and is aware of how the splint will feel (it's worth showing them a demo version).

  Lastly, make sure you have communicated to the patient what the treatment involves, especially how the splint will look and feel in their mouth, and what post-operative care will look like.

  It's important to show your patients some examples first. You don't want them to be shocked when you give them a chunky piece of plastic to hold! Therefore, make sure they know how it's going to look and feel when they use it.

Let us discuss the steps involved in making the splint.

Fabricating the michigan/tanner appliance

There are three steps involved in the process: a record taking step, a laboratory step and Michigan splint fit step.

- At the beginning of the first step, you're going to include **impressions**, an upper and lower arch, a **facebow record** and an **inter-occlusal record** in CR at a space of 2 mm from the first point of contact, leaving a minimum 2mm space for the splint. Therefore, when you open up the patient in CR at 2mm from CO, your splint is going to be, at minimum, 2mm thick.

- **In the laboratory a technician will:**
  - Mount the model in CR.
  - Wax it up.
  - Process the splint.
  - Sometimes you have the option of the processed model being remounted again, to check for some more guidance and make sure that the contacts are refined as shown in ***Figure 11***.

FIGURE 11

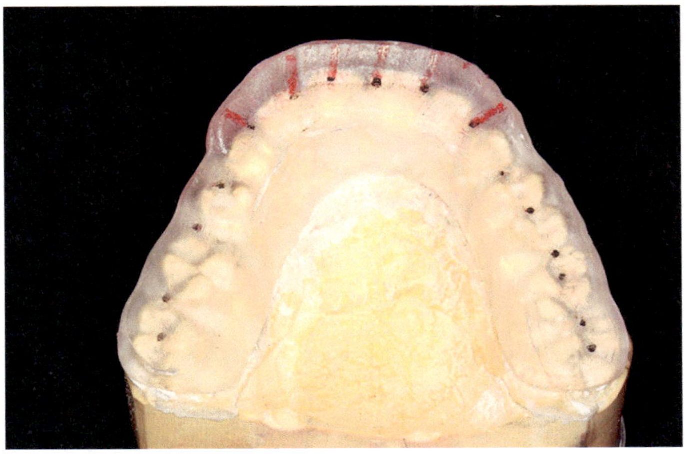

You may need to do some adjustments when a patient comes to see you to have the splint fitted, but if you have done all the checks accurately, they will likely be very minor.

- **When you see a patient for a clinical procedure:**
  - You're going to fit and adjust the splint as we discussed. Make sure that you assess the contact points and adjust this splint as necessary.
  - Review the patient for two consecutive appointments at maybe one or two weeks apart, until there is no change in contacts.
  - When you assess the patient a week later, make sure that the contacts are the same as what you provided them with at the fitting appointment.
  - You will often need to assess this either because the patient has not been using the splint or because you found CR the first time around and the patient's muscles were relaxed from the beginning.
  - Ultimately you want two consecutive appointments where the contacts and the guidance haven't changed from the ideal occlusion you had created, meaning you won't need to do any adjustments.

Let us look at these steps more in detail.

Clinical requirements for the construction of a maxillary occlusal splint

It's important to consider what the laboratory will require from you to construct a maxillary occlusal splint. You will need:

- Accurate impressions of the upper and lower maxillary case studies.
- The facebow record.
- The inter-occlusal record taken using an anterior deprogrammer.

These should help you mount high-quality maxillary and mandibular casts based on a true anatomical relationship on a semi-adjustable articulator (even though we all know and understand the limits of articulators or semi-adjustable articulators).

1.6 Facebow Records

In this chapter we are going to discuss facebow records. ***Figure 12*** shows various components of facebows.

FIGURE 12

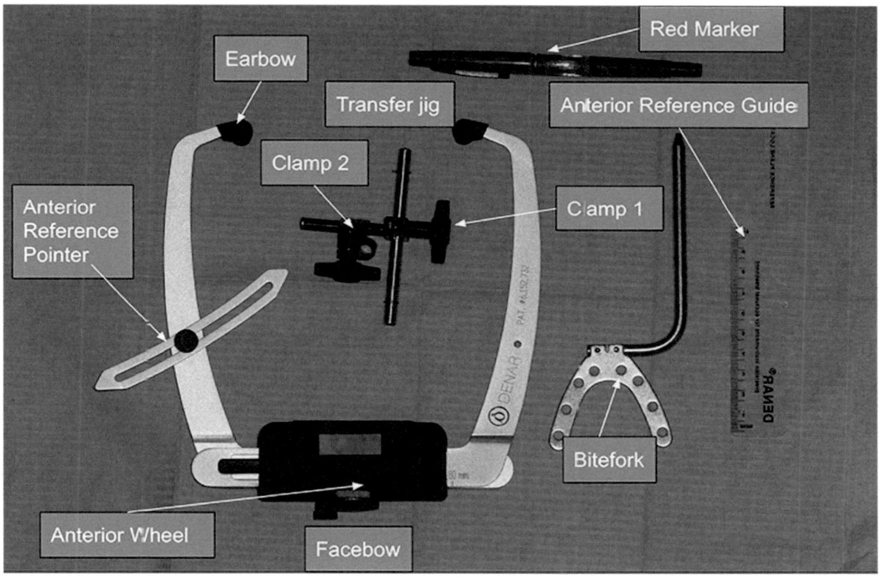

Facebow – why?

A facebow record is used to record the physical relationship between the maxilla and the occlusal surfaces of maxillary teeth, both in relation to the intercondylar hinge axis of the mandible and the horizontal plane.

A facebow helps with mounting models that depict an accurate replica of the patient's jaw movement. This can assist with:

- ❖ Assessment and treatment planning cases.
- ❖ A comprehensive and functional diagnostic wax up.

- Full mouth reconstruction cases where we need to mount patients' models in accurate positions.
- Incorporating or changing guidance in a restoration.

If you would like to change canine guidance, group function or incorporate protrusive guidance, it is best to mount models using a facebow.

- It also helps with mounting models when you're doing a complete denture.
- If a patient has an anterior open bite, then mounting models using a facebow gets you more accurate results because there are no anterior teeth to provide protrusive guidance and hence posterior teeth will have to provide all the guidance.
- It further helps you to record a patient's jaw relationship when you're fabricating a Michigan splint or a Tanner appliance.
- When you are restoring an upper second molar (let's say a posterior most tooth and especially a second molar), I would recommend mounting a model using a facebow because you need a very accurate position of the teeth, and because these models are not mounted often, many times when you see crowns coming back, usually they have high contact point. Because when you look at the arch and the closure of the jaw, any small discrepancy on the posterior teeth will exaggerate in the anterior aspect.
- So, make sure that when you're restoring posteriors, especially the last single standing tooth, you mount your models.

Functions of a facebow

- So in summary
- A facebow helps with orienting your maxillary models to the terminal hinge axis and the floor of the horizontal plane.
- It also helps in transferring the interocclusal plane so that it is aligned with the interpupillary line.
- Furthermore, it helps with mounting models centrally within the articulator.
- It allows for a reproducible transfer.

The fact that it allows for a reproducible transfer is the main reason I use a facebow. There are a lot of theories out there suggesting that you don't really need a facebow; yet a great benefit is that it allows me to mount models in a reproducible manner for any patient.

Therefore, if I'm doing a full mouth reconstruction case, I might mount models at different stages and want all those stages to be accurate for that patient. For that purpose, a facebow can be very good at providing reliable mounting.

- It also allows for a **maxillary cast verification.**
- A facebow will let you **measure the intercondylar distance**, although again, not all facebows do that. However, this may also not be entirely useful if your articulator has a fixed condylar distance.

Types of facebow

So what are the different types of facebow?

Kinematic facebow

If you want to measure a patient's true terminal hinge axis, then this is the best type of facebow, used for mounting a fully adjustable articulator.

However, a disadvantage is that it is time consuming and expensive, and it is a sensitive technique. It can only be used with fully adjustable articulators.

For most cases you do not need a fully adjustable articulator and I would argue you don't even need a semi-adjustable one. Most of the time you will need an average value articulator to do almost 50% of your full mouth reconstruction work.

Arbitrary facebow

There is another type of facebow called arbitrary facebow (***Figure 13***), one which assumes a few parameters and will make your life easier!

FIGURE 13

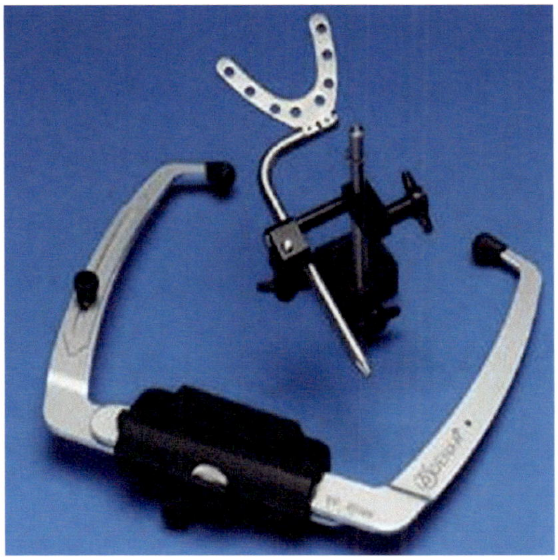

There are two main types of arbitrary facebows.

a) Facial type - Hanau 132-25m/132-2c
b) Earpiece type - Whipmix, Bergstrom, Denar slidematic

Denar's slidematic facebow is featured on the above photograph (***Figure 13***), and it assumes that the terminal hinge axis is approximately 13mm from the external auditory meatus, with a roughly 75% accuracy rate (so +/- 6mm).

Although this is arguably the best we have, it's not accurate. Therefore, we need to understand why it's called an arbitrary facebow, as it assumes some of those parameters.

Kois analyser

This is for when you're doing aesthetic cases and you want to have the occlusal plane just right. The denar slidematic facebow does record that, but the Kois is the best at recording the occlusal plane and the interpupillary line for aesthetic cases.

Facebow components

We are going to look at the denar slidematic facebow (***Figure 14***) in more detail in this section, including its components.

FIGURE 14

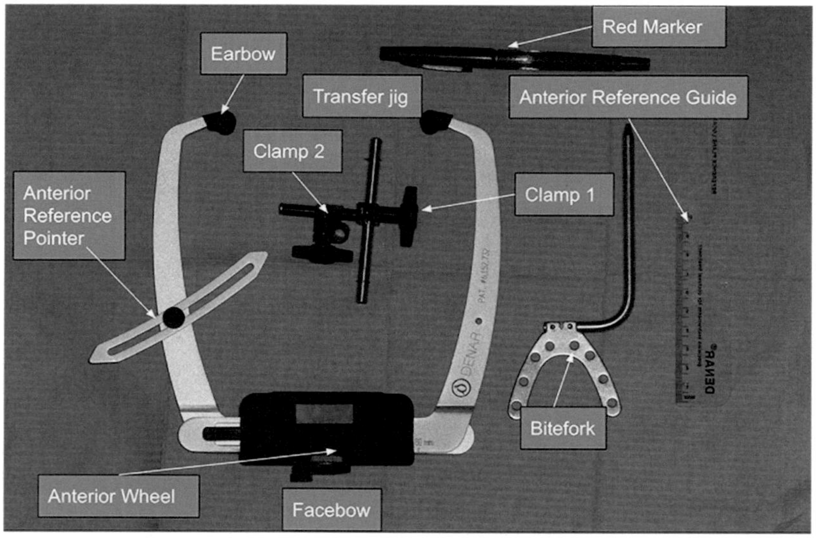

You will need a bite fork, a mounting platform, and the transfer jig with clamp. You will also have the anterior reference guide (set at 43mm), as well as the anterior wheel, the anterior reference pointer and the earbow.

Facebow record instructions

Step by step procedure:

- Mark the **anterior reference point** on the right side of the nose using a denar ruler from the midpoint of the incisal edge of UR2 (43mm). If there is missing UR2 then use UR1 or UR3 , if all teeth are missing then use the lower border of the upper lip.
- Assess the size of the maxillary arch (length and width). If the bite fork does not fit well then modify the bite fork with an impression compound or putty.
- Choose the recording medium for the bite fork - the impression compound, bite reg or moyco beauty wax (hard wax). I will describe the technique needed for the bite reg material below:
    1. Dispense the first 1cm of material and then inject vertically onto the bite fork, ensuring that the material has extruded through the holes on the bite fork for retention purposes.
    2. Use your finger to swipe against the material to make a flat surface.
    3. Place in the mouth gently, ensuring that the midline coincides with the midline mark on the bite fork. Make sure it's in the center from both sides and not tilted anterior-posteriorly. Apply gentle pressure to get only the light indentations as shown in figure 12b.
    4. Check the indents – you want shallow indents of the cusp tips.
    5. Trim the deep areas (with a scalpel no.11 blade or acrylic bur if material allows) and remove the areas of deep fissure and only leave cusp indentations. For this to work, the bite reg material needs to be thick.
    6. Place the maxillary cast onto the bite fork material and check to see if the cast is stable. Check that all the cusp tips on the maxillary cast can fit into the indentations made. Make sure it matches the same as what you can see in the mouth. Aim to capture at least the last standing tooth and anterior teeth to get tripod type contacts for better stability of the model.

- Ask the patient to hold the bite fork in place on the maxillary teeth.
- Ensure all the screw components of the earbow and transfer jig are loose (except the anterior reference pointer on the earbow).
- Place the earbow earplug components into the ears and ask the patient to indicate the fit and comfort.

- Tighten the middle screw to lock the intercondylar distance.
- Attach the transfer jig #2 clamp hole to the arm of the bite fork.
- Attach the vertical shaft of the transfer jig to the earbow. Ensure it is fully seated into the earbow before tightening the screw.
- Align the anterior reference pointer to mark the nose and tighten the screw.
- Check the horizontal alignment of the earbow to the interpupillary line and tighten the screw clamp 1.
- Slightly pull the transfer jig to allow the earplug components to move anteriorly and tighten screw clamp 2.
- Re-check the alignment of the earbow and jig and check the tightness of the screws. Make sure you see no 21 when you look at the clamps 1 and 2.
- Release the middle screw, widen the ear components and remove the bite fork to release the patient from the whole set up.
- Release the earbow from the transfer jig.
- Disinfect the assembly and package it in a rigid box before sending it to the laboratory.

Make sure when you're using the **facebow** that it is parallel to both the interpupillary line and the floor.

Figure 15a and ***Figure 15b*** show different materials, impression compound and rigid bite registration material for the bitefork. Note shallow indentations. ***Figure 15c*** and ***Figure 15d*** show a mounted maxillary model.

FIGURE 15a

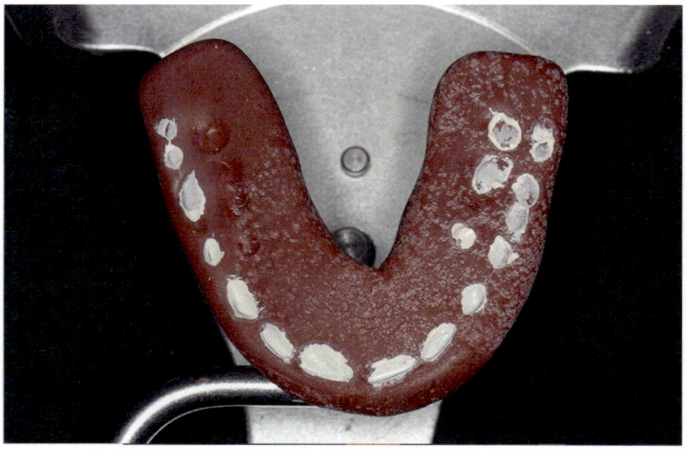

FIGURE 15b

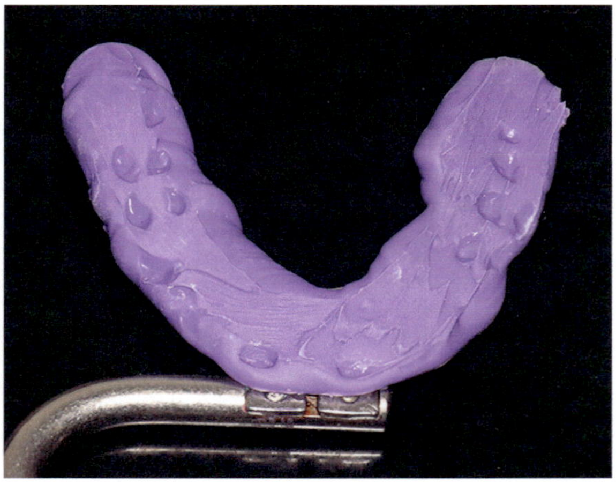

FIGURE 15c

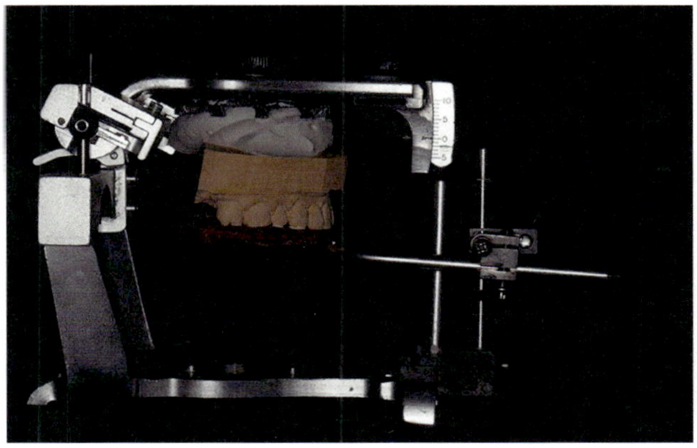

FIGURE 15d

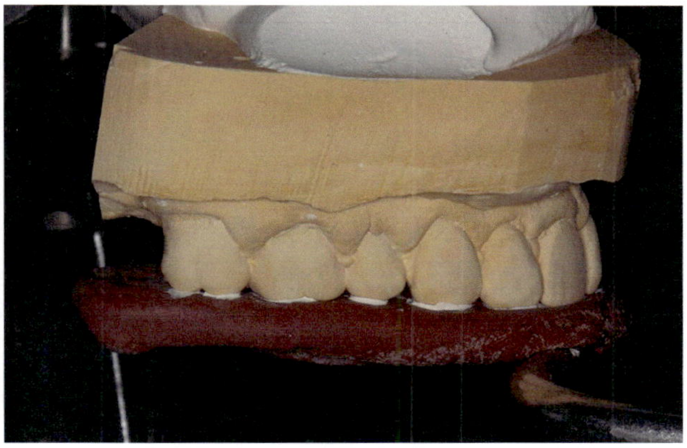

Facebow – tips

As you can see in ***Figure 16***, if you look from the side, the **facebow** is parallel to the interpupillary line, but the fork is not really parallel to the floor. Therefore there is a bit of a discrepancy. **Figure 17** shows the same photo from a different angle.

FIGURE 16

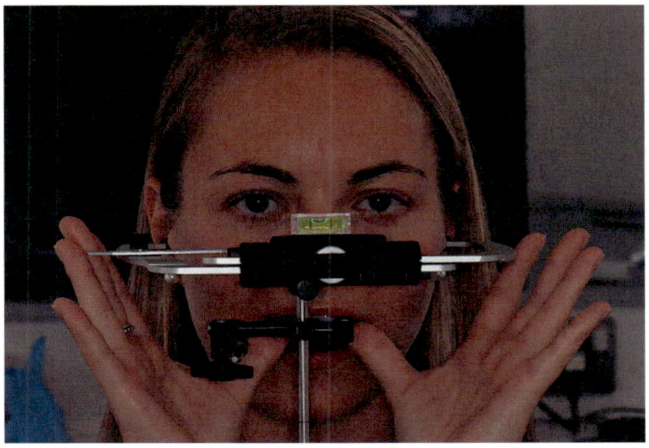

FIGURE 17

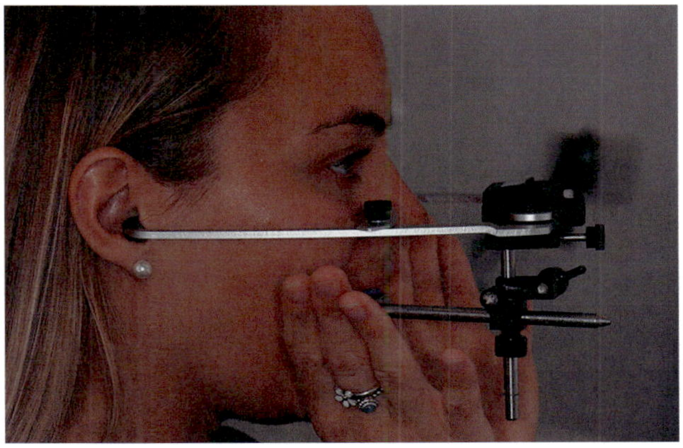

So just remember when you're starting with a facebow, **you will need to create a small dot** as a third reference point as shown in ***Figure 18a***.

<u>FIGURE 18a</u>

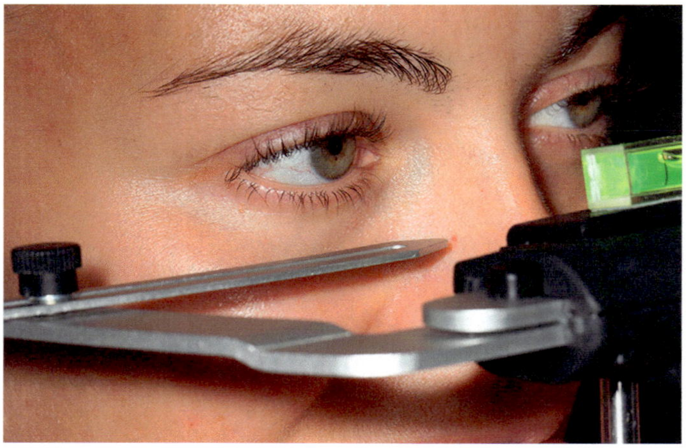

You will see that on the facebow you have a marker leveler on top. You don't really need to use that leveler all the time because it depends on the angulation of the patient's head. The air bubble can go either side, so the leveler is not really entirely reliable.

- **Use the incisal edge of the lateral incisor to mark an arbitrary reference point of around 43 mm with a ruler.**
  If the patient doesn't have a lateral incisor then use a central incisor.

  If a patient has no teeth then use the upper lip, with the lower border of the upper lip as a reference point. This is not really ideal, as you cannot use the patient's ridge as a reference point.

- **Make sure the fork is straight and not tilted.**
  If the midline has not shifted, then you can take the midline as the reference to align the notch on the bite fork. So as we discussed, your bite fork notch needs to coincide with the midline as shown on ***Figure 18b.***

  Now what if the midline has shifted? In that case, you cannot take the midline as the reference point to align the notch on the bite. You can use the frenum or center line of the face instead, recording the midline shift and making sure it matches what's in your articulator.

- **Make sure you have the handle of the bite fork on the right side of the patient as shown in *Figure 18b*** and ***18c.***

FIGURE 18b

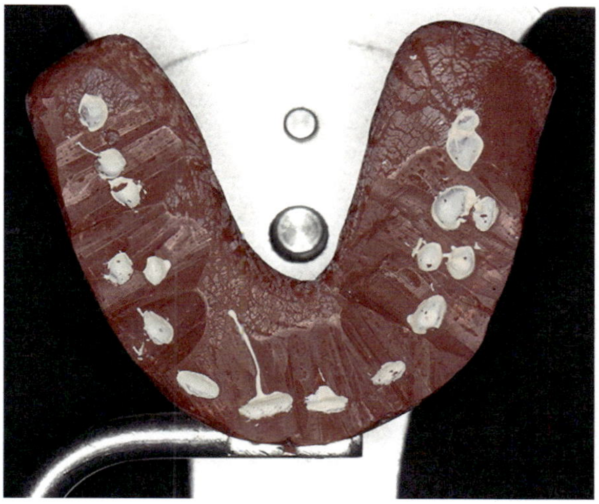

FIGURE 18c

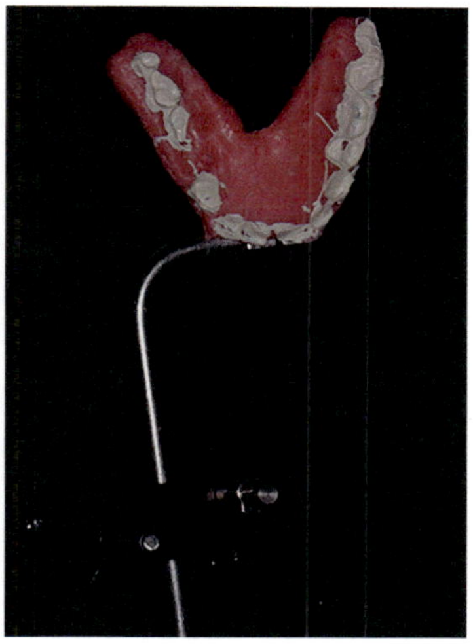

Again, this is a very important detail as it means the bite fork is the correct way up. Many dentists end up using bite forks the other way around, so just make sure that it's on the right side of the patient.

- **You can just use three points (two most posterior points on either side and one anterior point) on the bite fork to capture the arch.**
  This is because all we want is our maxillary cast to be stable. Sometimes if you're using the material in a full arch, you might find it difficult to locate the jig and might be risking it by pushing it too far inwards and creating a big indentation.

  If you want, you can just use three points with the posterior tooth on each side and some anterior teeth. Those three points will still stabilise the model.

  However, using more teeth is preferable for assuring the stability of the model.

- **Again, remember once you tighten number 1 and then number 2 clamps it should look like a number 21 and make sure the jig is fully seated into the earbow.**
  Many times when I'm teaching a dentist how to do a facebow record they don't tighten the jig fully, which means it is not fully seated into the facebow earpiece assembly. You need to make sure it is nicely and fully seated and tightened up so it doesn't move before you start recording the facebow.

You need to make sure that the number you have is 21, as shown in the photo (***Figure 19***).

FIGURE 19

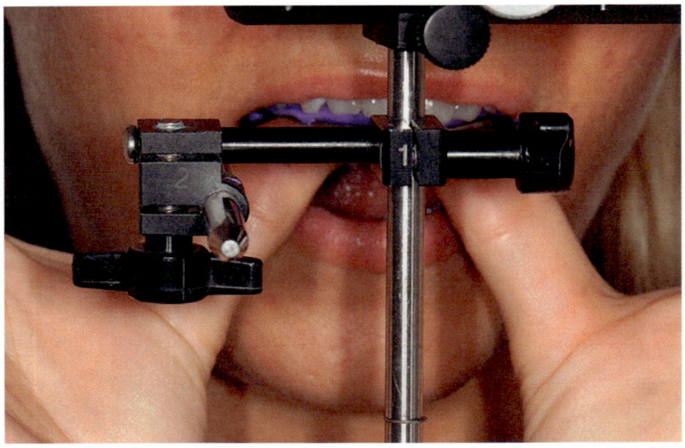

You can see number two and one, although if you tighten number one first and then two, it looks like 21. This is very important.

❖ **Furthermore, don't forget to pull the earbow before tightening number two.**

❖ **Check to see if the ears are parallel.**
This is very important because sometimes the ears are not at the same level, and when you put on the earbow you won't be able to get the interpupillary line straight.

In this case, what you can do is take the earpiece out from the relevant ear and move it a little bit upward or downward because we want the interpupillary line to be stable rather than the ears to be aligned.

I would therefore consider adjusting the earpieces so that they are aligned, even if one of them is not in the ear. Because the layout of the face can be arbitrary, you may have to accept that it may not be that accurate.

❖ **Keep the patient upright when you're tightening the transfer jig, as it really helps when taking your records.**
For the bite fork, you can keep the patient lying down because that helps with gaining access. If you're tightening everything and checking the interpupillary line, then it's better if you keep the patient upright so that you can look at the level of the floor compared with the interpupillary line and get the best record.

- **Make sure that both arms of the facebow are parallel to the floor. If they aren't, then you can lose the number one clamp, make the facebow parallel and then tighten the clamp again.**

  This should sort the problem out. So, make sure to look at this in a three-dimensional way and ensure it's nice and stable all the way around.

  Furthermore, make sure that screws one and two are tightened properly and take the whole assembly out from the facebow, before the jig. Make sure you let the nurse know, if they are new, not to dismantle your record.

1.7 Inter Occlusal Records

When might you need interocclusal records?

- If you would like to **mount models in CR or CO**, you will need interocclusal records. If you are doing full mouth reconstruction and if you're going to increase OVD, then you need the teeth to be apart and that's when we use inter-occlusal records.

  If you're increasing the OVD, you cannot use the current teeth as guidance because once you open the bite, there will be no reference for you to go back to once you start restoring teeth.

- Another time you would use inter-occlusal records is when a patient is unable to close their teeth in one stable position. In other words, if the **bite is unstable,** you will need interocclusal records. Even if you're planning to mount a model in ICP and the patient's bite is not stable, you may still need an interocclusal record. To make sure that the models are stabilised or if the patient has lost many teeth, then you still need some sort of interocclusal record.

- **Fabrication of the Michigan splint,** as we discussed previously, will also require you to take interocclusal records.

When you don't need interocclusal records

- You don't need them when the patient's occlusion is stable and your restorations do not involve a reorganised approach or an increase of OVD.
- Similarly, if you're mounting models in ICP then you don't really need interocclusal records as long as you are able to put together and locate both upper and lower models easily.

Remember: You always need a facebow record to mount any models. You just don't need interocclusal records if you don't want to mount the model in CR and the bite is stable.

Recording CR using different types of methods

You need to understand the various methods of recording CR before you choose which one is best for you.

- **Bimanual manipulation**

  We'll start with bimanual manipulation, taught at numerous universities and in my hands-on course. It is really helpful because when you're recording a bite you do need to be able to relax the patient.

  However, this is a very sensitive technique, and you cannot rely on it all the time, especially when you're doing bite registration as it's very difficult for a patient who is dysfunctional to be asked to stay open in one position while your material sets.

  So, although I use bimanual manipulation for my assessments, I don't use it for interocclusal records.

  When you're doing bimanual manipulation (***Figure 20***), make sure you have your thumbs in the patient's mouth just below the teeth for support while having three fingers on the angle of the mandible, rather than it digging into the floor of the mouth. Dentists often forget this, which means the hand slips and fingers start digging below the floor area of the mouth, which is uncomfortable for the patient. So, use the mandible as your support.

FIGURE 20

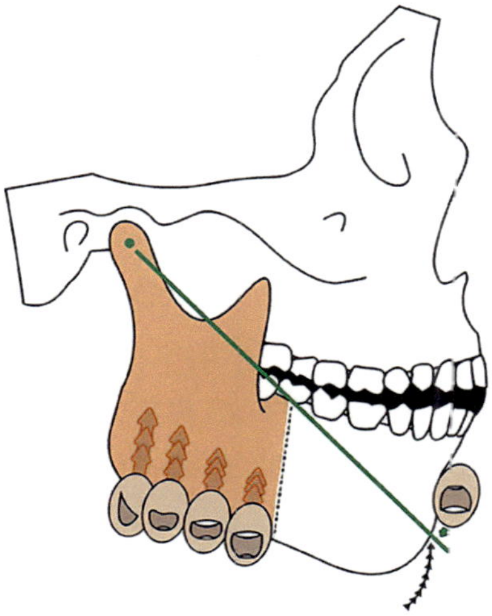

What you are trying to do is slot the condyle into the socket in the anterior superior position, guiding the patient's jaw and ultimately condyle. But as you can imagine, this is very difficult when patients are dysfunctional. If the patient is very relaxed, and there are no parafunctional habits going on, then it is simpler to use this technique.

Therefore, what I would suggest is that before you start using this technique in anyone dysfunctional, try and use it in younger patients who haven't yet damaged their teeth or muscles, as they are likely to be much more relaxed.

It requires a lot of practice, so make sure you do it!

❖ **Anterior deprogrammer**

One of my favorite deprogrammers is the **Lucia jig**. You can use any anterior deprogrammer to record interocclusal records. However, you need to make sure that the deprogrammer, while you're recording, is not covering the whole arch because you need to place some sort of a bite registration material to capture position.

The lucia jig only covers the front 2-3teeth, and because of that you will have posterior teeth which are not covered and you can use your interocclusal material easily to take the record.

Here are different types of anterior deprogrammers:

- Lucia Jig
- Leaf Gauge
- Kois Deprogrammer
- NTI-tss Splint
- Cranham Deprogrammer

Let's look at all of them one-by-one, starting with:

- ***Lucia jig***

  The lucia jig is fabricated by using either the DuraLay (***Figure 21***) or Bosworth's trim (acrylic resin) material. The benefit of making it from resin is that it provides a hard surface for the patient to close on and has an in-built stop point. You can adjust the height according to your needs and be able to mark the position.

  Therefore, when you're placing interocclusal material between the teeth, you are sure that the patient is closing in the most relaxed position, the one which you previously recorded and marked.

FIGURE 21

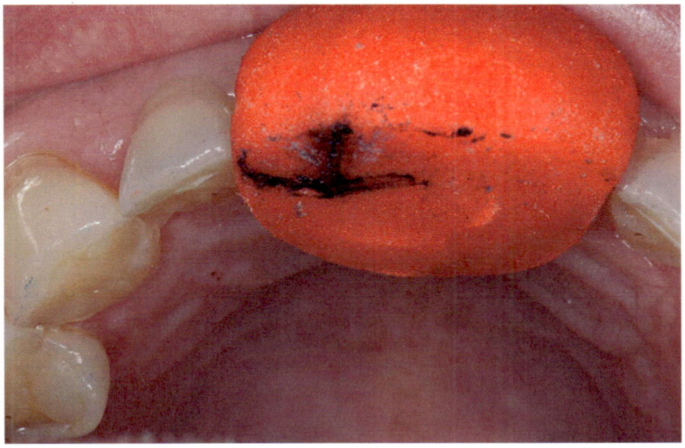

- ***Leaf gauge***
  *Leaf gauge (**Figure 22,** Huffman's leaf gauge)*
  1 Leaf = 0.1mm thickness

FIGURE 22

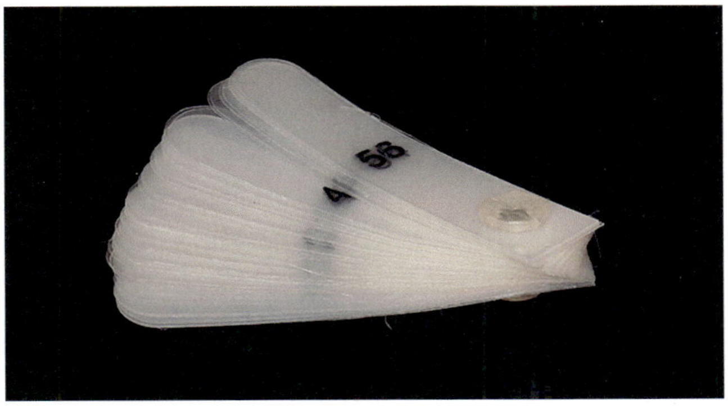

If you want something quicker than the leaf gauge is a quick and easy way to assess occlusion, which is also very helpful in recording interocclusal records.

This is my method of choice during occlusal assessment, load testing of TMJ and for finding CO.

To record an interocclusal record using a leaf gauge, ask the patient to grind on the gauge forwards and backwards a few times. Once you feel the patient's jaw has gone back far enough and is most relaxed, ask them to open their mouth and squeeze the bite registration material on the upper and lower teeth on both sides.

Then ask the patient to close on the leaf gauge and repeat the forwards and backwards movements just once. You can then support the patient's jaw in that position until the bite registration material sets.

- ***Kois deprogrammer***
  You can use the Kois deprogrammer when a patient has got a very dysfunctional joint, as it is very difficult to record their bite on the same appointment.

  So if a patient comes to see me and I can't get them to relax using a lucia jig or leaf gauge, then I might have to give them something to take home and use for a couple of weeks to relax their jaw and make sure it's deprogrammed properly, before bringing them back again to record the interocclusal record.

  It is not possible to use the lucia jig at home at night because it is too small, and there is a risk of inhalation particularly at night. The Kois deprogrammer is very effective if you want to give patients something temporary for a couple of weeks before you record that position.

  However, if the patient is very dysfunctional, consider giving them a Michigan splint because it can be used for long term without any issues.

- ***NTI-tss splint***
  You also can use the NTI-tss appliance, which is like a prefabricated version of the lucia jig. You just need to reline it from the inside before you use it.

- ***Cranham deprogrammer***
  The Cranham deprogrammer is another device which the patient can take home.This doesn't cover the patient's teeth. It only covers the palate, and because of that you can use it while you are doing an interocclusal record, particularly after the patient has relaxed with it at home.

Materials used to record interocclusal records

Figure 23 shows the various materials used for interocclusal records.

FIGURE 23

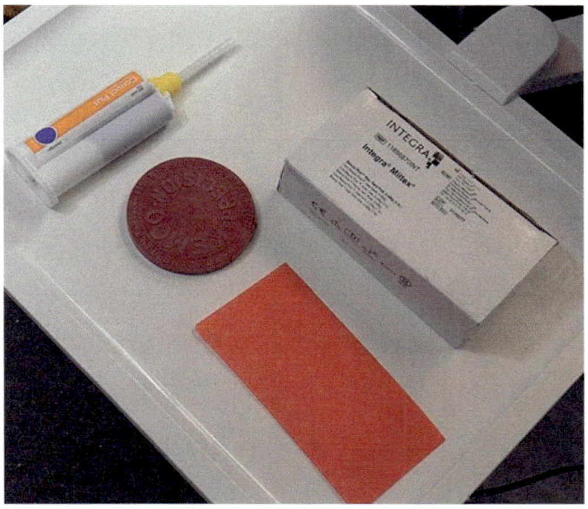

- **You can use hard bite registration material** such as Moyco Beauty wax which sets really hard and is brittle. You don't want anything soft and springy! Be aware that the Moyco beauty wax is not the same as the pink wax.It is a special wax that becomes brittle at room temperature. It only becomes soft when you are heating it up.
- Another possibility is a good hard bite registration material which is rigid and easy to trim.

A step-by-step guide for fabrication of the Lucia jig:

- Use vaseline on the teeth on which you will be making Lucia jig. You can premake the Lucia jig using study models and then reline it in the patient's mouth.
- Prepare and mix the acrylic.
- At the doughy stage, place the mixture over the central incisors. Avoid an overextension on the mucosa as it will be time-consuming to adjust once it's set and it will give unnecessary feedback to the patient which can affect recording CR. Use a spatula to make the palatal surface of the jig flat. Make sure this is at a slight angle replicating gentle incline of the palatal surface. However, make sure it's not too steep otherwise it will force the mandible into a retruded position which is not ideal.
- Manipulate the patient and allow them to close together so that the OVD is at an ideal level as per your assessment. You can use composite for a mock up to evaluate the ideal increase of OVD. Measure this increase using gingival zenith of the upper and lateral incisors as a reference and when you are making Lucia jig make sure you are at the same OVD.

- Check the setting of the acrylic and heat it has generated. Gently remove and reseat so as not to overheat the teeth and to avoid the jig locking into the undercuts. If needed, place the jig in the cold water for a couple of seconds. Be aware not to leave it out for too long otherwise it will not seat again due to shrinkage.
- Trim the palatal surface to remove the incisal indentations and make a flat platform with acrylic bur or a model trimmer.
- Check the stability and retention of the jig. Reline if needed with an acrylic or a silicone bite reg material.
- Manipulate the patient and check the retruded point of contact on the jig (mark in black).
- Check the forward and backward movements. Use black articulating paper to mark the line.
- Once this has been established, you can use flowable composite on the jig to capture the most retruded position, so you can relocate this back after placement of inter occlusal material.

Step by step protocol for recording CR using Moyco beauty wax:

- Soften the moyco beauty wax in warm water and fold over to get double thickness.
- Make indents of the maxillary teeth intraorally or by using the existing study cast.
- Cut the anterior portion into a V shape (incisor areas) to allow space for the lucia jig. Fold over the cut area, sealing and folding the corners over the canines. Cut the rest of the excess using buccal cusp tips as a guide. Also remove any excess distal on the last tooth. Seal the edges using a heated instrument. You can reinforce the wax by using aluminum foil in-between. However, this is not necessary.
- Insert the lucia jig as fabricated above.
- Warm the wax template and place over the maxillary teeth.
- Guide/manipulate the patient into CR and allow them to close through the wax onto the lucia jig. Check that it has made contact with the retruded mark on the jig.
- Remove the lucia jig and allow the patient to squeeze more into the wax (creating a space for the Temp-Bond) but making sure the patient does not go through the wax completely. Check that the wax template has not been grossly distorted or perforated in many places.
- Chill the wax template in cold water.
- Place the lucia jig and wax template back in the mouth. Ask the patient to close on the lucia jig and check to see some movement of the template. This will confirm that extra space has been created for the Temp-Bond.
- Remove the wax template from the mouth. Dry the template. Mix the Temp-Bond and place on the mandibular side of the wax template in cusp tips.

- Guide/manipulate the patient into CR and allow the patient to close through the Temp-Bond onto the lucia jig. Check that it is contacting onto the retruded mark on the jig (the Temp-Bond will fill the space that was created in the wax template when the patient squeezed).
- Allow the Temp-Bond to set and remove the wax template and lucia jig.
- Trim with the No.11 scalpel blade any excess/unsupported/deep fissure areas of Temp-Bond.

When you are taking an interocclusal record, make sure you take more than one. That way when you mount the models, you can then verify that your records match.

Figure 24a shows lucia jig with markings.
Figure 24b shows three interocclusal records of the same patient.

FIGURE 24a

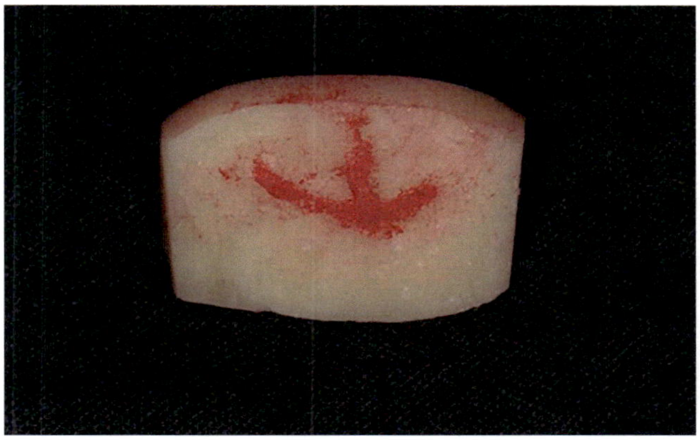

FIGURE 24b

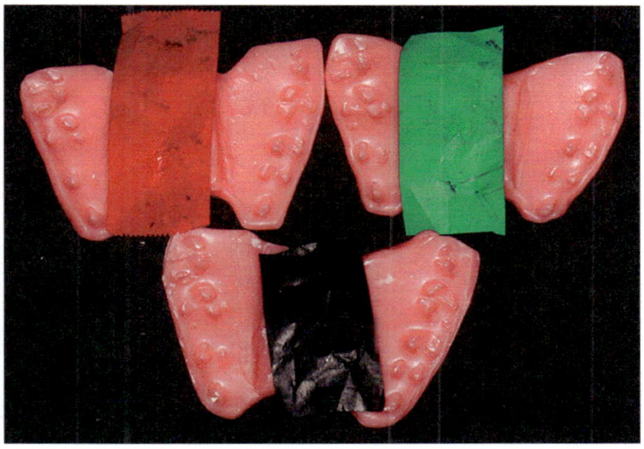

Figure 24c shows mounting of the model in CR using interocclusal records.
Figure 24d shows Denar Vericheck to check accuracy of three interocclusal records.

FIGURE 24c

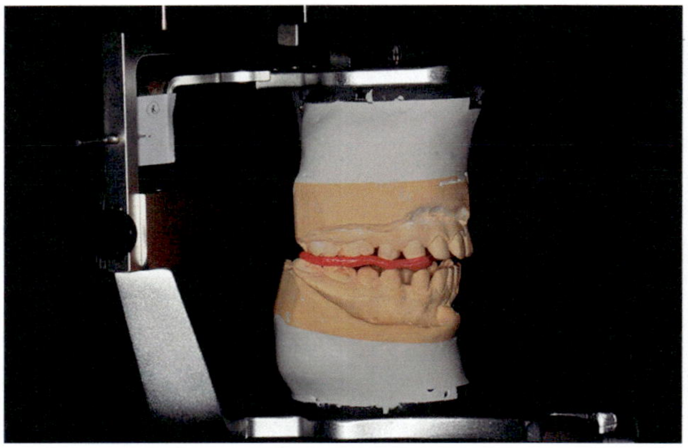

FIGURE 24d

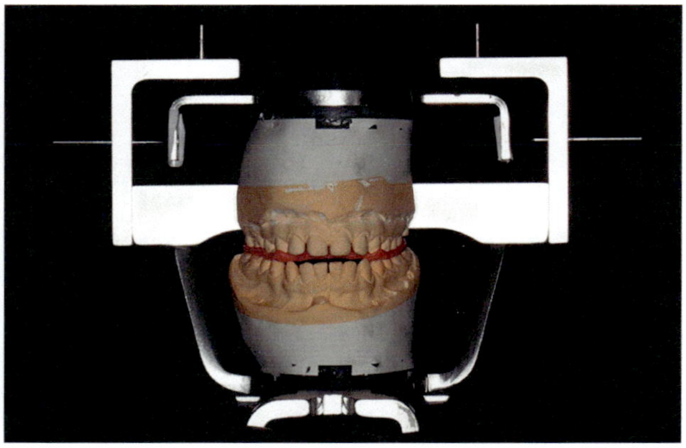

FIGURES 24e and ***24f*** show the Denar Vericheck to check accuracy of three interocclusal records showing three dots in different colours overlapping each other showing perfect match.

FIGURE 24e

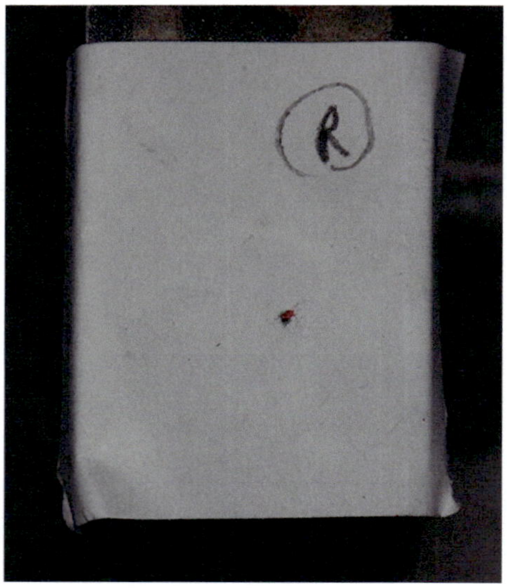

FIGURE 24f

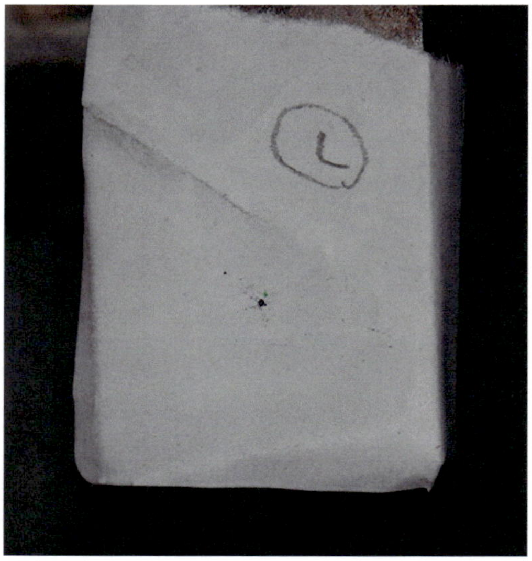

If you mount two sets of models you will know whether your records are accurate or not.

It's also worth checking the first point of contact after mounting models. Let's say I've mounted some models and once I've dropped the pin, if my first point of contact is the same as what I found in the mouth, then I know that my records are accurate.

Alternative interocclusal material:

- If you feel the above technique is too complex then you can use hard bite registration material instead. Simply ask the patient to open the mouth, place lucia jig as fabricated above and squeeze bite registration material on both sides and ask the patient to close the jaw on the lucia jig and guide the patient into the relaxed position marked previously.

Step by step protocol for recording CR using Leaf gauge

- Place leaf gauge in between the front teeth and position the patient into CR by asking the patient to repeatedly move their jaw forwards and backwards.
- Ask the patient to open their mouth and insert bite registration material on the back teeth.
- Place the leaf gauge back and ask the patient to go forward and backward just once.
- While the patient is moving backwards, guide the patient into CR and support the jaw.
- Once material is set, adjust the bite reg to remove any deep fissure impressions and make sure only cusp tips indentations have remained to ensure complete seating of the models.

As you can see, using a leaf gauge is a very easy process. However, you need to make sure that the bite registration material you use is a hard material and does not flex.

How thick should the interocclusal record be?

Many dentists ask me how thick their interocclusal record needs to be, how thick the lucia jig needs to be, and how many leaves need to be in the leaf gauge**.** The thickness of your occlusal record depends on whether you're using the Michigan splint for diagnostic reasons or for restorative reasons.

Here is a quick guide on recommended thickness for each clinical scenario:

Diagnostic:

- **CO (appropriate thickness to capture first point of contact).**
- **Mounting in CR (teeth should be apart but as little as possible).**

If you're using it for diagnostic reasons, then you need to mount the model in a centric occlusion, or as minimum opening in CR as possible.

Therefore, you need to make sure that if you are recording a patient's CR for diagnostic purposes, you want the opening to be as minimal as possible - the reason being that when you are mounting a model on an articulator, you want to avoid opening and closing the pin on the articulator because we know that unless you use a fully adjustable articulator, you will not be able to replicate the movement exactly as it was in the mouth.

All articulators have some inaccuracies, and so won't open or close exactly like your mouth or your patient's mouth. Therefore, the idea is to mount the model in the correct vertical position so that you don't have to open or close it in the articulator.

This is why mounting in CO is very straightforward, but mounting in CR for diagnostic purposes will mean you want to keep the gap as small as possible.

Michigan splint

- **2mm opening from CO.**
  If you are using interocclusal records for a Michigan splint then as we discussed, you will need a 2mm space from the CO to get the required level of thickness.

Restorative

- **Amount of increase in OVD.**
- **Aesthetics needs.**
- **Depends on if you are mounting in CO or CR.**

If you're using it for treatment purposes, then you need to have the right amount of thickness to replicate the amount of increase in OVD.

This is something you can try by just doing some composite mockups in a patient's mouth, building some direct composite without any bond, to check and assess the vertical dimension you need. Remember to mount the models or keep the interocclusal record thick enough to provide you with restorative space.

Another factor is aesthetics. Again, do a mockup of the anterior teeth as it will tell you what type of aesthetics you're looking at and the increase in OVD you need.

It will also depend on whether you're doing a restorative case using CO or CR. With the above situation, where you're mounting a model and increasing the OVD for aesthetic purposes, you'll most likely be mounting a model in CR.

If you are using your CO as your restorative space creator, then it's very straightforward to mount the model in CO and have the interocclusal records replicated. However, you will be limited to working in the space you have created, and will have to fit into this space by opening in CO.

I hope now you now know the importance of the Michigan splint when it comes to occlusion and full mouth reconstruction. It is important to understand the exact process of fitting it properly. In the next chapter we will discuss the steps involved in fitting the Michigan splint.

1.8 Understanding of Fitting and Adjusting of the Michigan Splint

Before fitting and adjusting

Before fitting and adjusting a Michigan Splint make sure to:

- **Minimise any clinical errors in both clinical and laboratory procedures.**
  Before we discuss fitting and adjusting the Michigan splint, it is very important that you understand the importance of minimising any clinical and laboratory errors in fabricating the splint.

- **Use a laboratory with a high standard of precision.**
  Therefore, use the best laboratory with the highest standards of best practice when you are sending in your work. To make them understand the specification, you may have to be very prescriptive. Inform the technician that you would like a shallow guidance, lateral guidance provided by canine and protrusive guidance by centrals and laterals.

  Often technicians make the anterior ramp very steep in order to get posterior disclusion, which might make their life easier but will be wrong for the patient as it may lock their occlusion. It's very difficult to create a nice, shallow anterior guidance on the splint while still keeping the posterior disclusion and making sure that you have a splint that is workable. Hence, you need a technician who takes extra care in fabricating the splint.

Fitting an occlusal splint

Fitting the splint can be broken down into two steps:

Step 1: assess the fit of the device.
Step 2: adjust it to gain optimal contact.

Step 1: Assessing and refining the quality of fit

So, let's look at step one, where we will assess and refine the quality of the fit.

Make sure that the precision and comfort levels are right. Make sure there is positive seating under gentle pressure, as you don't want any active pressure when you're seating the splint. You want some passivity, but you also want enough retention for the splint to stay on.

An undercut can be removed or adjusted in the splint to make sure that it's not active but retentive. So, if a technician has not blocked those big undercuts, causing patients to feel pain, then it needs to be adjusted.

Many times when you fit their splint, the patient will feel that the anterior teeth are a bit tight. It's very common because of the arc of rotation, and when you're fitting the splint, the way the anterior teeth are placed means you do not have a perfect fit. Hence, an adjustment will be needed especially when a technician has created some overlap.

Silicone impression material or pressure-indicating paste may be used to check the pressure points if the splint is not fitting properly. You can use light body silicone material for the splint and place the splint in the patient's mouth and check. You can also use occlusal indicator sprays. If the fit is wrong, then ideally you need to start again as otherwise step two will be redundant.

Sometimes you can salvage the splint by just creating a big trench and inserting acrylic resin, realigning the splint in the patient's mouth. Although this does solve the immediate problem, in the long run the splint becomes unhygienic and quickly breaks down internally. That's why it's not recommended.

However, you can realign one or two teeth. Let's say you have made a patient a Michigan splint and then the patient needed some indirect restoration or a change in the shape of the teeth. You can realign them after you've done the restoration. So it's ok for a few teeth but trenching the whole splint is not really ideal especially if it's new.

Of course, if it's an old splint and the patient wants to save money by not having the new one, you may use this as a temporary solution. However, you will need to let your patient know that it's a temporary solution, not a permanent one.

Step 2: Adjustment of the splint to gain optimal occlusal contacts

Now you can move on to step two, which covers the adjustment for the optimal occlusal contacts.

Many splints become ineffective because they have not been adjusted properly. Dentists often just give patients splints without adjustment. Unfortunately, in these circumstances the splint doesn't do what it's supposed to do and gains a bad reputation.

Therefore, make sure that initially you take time when you're adjusting the occlusal splint. Don't go overboard, as any appointment longer than 45 minutes will be counterproductive, but instead make sure you adjust as much as you can in that time.

If you cannot get the contact to be perfect, then take a break as if you carry on you will tire the patient out, compromising your ability to get a good result. Let the patient go with the splint in, see them again in two or three days, and reassess the contact points and adjust them again.

Make sure that you correctly adjust the splint, checking the contact point with a GHM articulating paper (12 microns thick), or you can use shim stock to check the contact points and make sure that the final adjustment is done.

Once you've done the final adjustment of the splint, you are looking for three criteria.

In the CR position, there should be **at least one holding point of contact per mandibular tooth**. So, if a patient has 14 mandibular teeth then make sure you get at least 14 contacts, with one contact per tooth on your splint. If you get two or three contacts, then that's fine. But just make sure it's a point contact, not a big smudge.

Make sure that once the patient has the splint fitted and is closing their mouth the teeth make contact everywhere, but the anterior contacts are light. Posterior contacts can be a little bit heavier, but anterior contacts need to be light.

In protrusive mode, you need to make sure that the **guidance is shallow but with immediate posterior disclusion**. So you're not keeping the anterior ramp really steep – instead you are having a shallow anterior ramp but with immediate posterior disclusion.

With lateral excursion, you are obviously using **canine guidance**, so make sure the mandibular posterior teeth lift instantly, as soon as the patient moves laterally. So essentially, we are trying to mimic the mutually protected occlusion or concepts of mutually protected occlusion within your Michigan splint.

Instructions for patient

Now that you have fitted and adjusted Michigan splint, you need to give your patient the appropriate instructions.

- **The patient should be instructed on the correct seating and removal of the splint.** They should expect some discomfort in the beginning, so ask them to ignore it for a couple of weeks unless it's very severe.

- **You also need to let the patient know how long you want them to wear the splint for.** If patients wear a Michigan splint for the whole day, initially it will help them. However, in the long run, they'll get used to it and then their muscle problem will return.

  So, you want intermittent use from the patient. However, if it's for protection of a restoration, then the patient must use it every night to protect them. But you need to guide them as to how long depending on the clinical needs.

- **Proper hygiene of the splint is very important because it can otherwise become a place that harbours bacteria.** Therefore, you need to make sure you give them hygiene instructions.

- **You need to provide a case with storage instructions. I usually tell patients to keep them dry (you don't need to put them in water like dentures), and keep them away from radiators or any heating source.**

Follow up

- Make sure that you see the patient for a follow-up in a couple of days to make sure everything is fine.
- After that you're going to see them on a weekly basis until there are no issues with the occlusal contact points. Once you give patients a Michigan splint, there can be rapid changes in muscle tone.
- Once you assess a patient for two consecutive appointments and there are no changes, you can assume that the muscles are in the most relaxed position possible.
- Having said that, some patients will not wear their splint. That's why I use a marker pen to make marks on the splint, as if a patient is using it, you can see the scratches over the marks replicating their grinding pattern and contact points. If they aren't, then the articulating paper marks will still be there.
- If all is well after two consecutive appointments, you can let the patient go and review them every six months or yearly.

Make sure that when you are assessing a patient after two weeks that you are watching for the right outcomes. Let's look at those outcomes in more detail.

Outcomes and implications

❖ Patient's level of comfort

Increased comfort suggests:

- **Occlusal factors are playing a role in TMD** for that patient. If patients feel better in their joints and muscles, that means their occlusion was playing a role in their TMD. By giving them a splint, you have changed their occlusion.
- **The patient is able to adapt to a new occlusal scheme**. If you're going to give patients a full mouth reconstruction or a full mouth of new restorations, they will most likely get used to changes more easily.
- **The possibility of a significant placebo effect** is there, as some patients will be cured because they feel that it's working.
- You get predictable results in these types of patients because **their adaptive capability is good.**

Poor tolerance and increased discomfort suggest:

- You need to consider either **a misdiagnosis** on your part, with the patient not having occlusal-related problems.
- ...or it could be that there is a very critical balance between occlusion and **a poor neuromuscular structure.** There are some patients who will not tolerate an increase in the OVD at all, and by giving them a Michigan splint, you may worsen their symptoms.
- It is desirable to resort to minimal occlusal intervention. So in these patients, you need to make sure that you're not doing any extensive treatment because they may be **unsuitable for extensive restorative treatment.**
- You may have to work with the existing dentition, and just try and keep those teeth until they change. Sometimes their neuromuscular structure changes, which means you could try again with a splint in the future.

❖ The amount of increase in the occlusal vertical relationship

As discussed previously, one of the reasons you would use the Michigan splint is to assess the patient's adaptive capabilities for a predefined increased OVD. If a patient can tolerate this easily then you can be assured that the patient may not have problems with increasing OVD at that level. And plan your full mouth reconstruction accordingly.

- **The presence of an identifiable occlusal slide**
  If the problem is localised and there is an identifiable occlusal slide, then it's easy to eliminate it after patients have used the Michigan splint because their muscles will be much more relaxed, and you can easily make adjustments in the patient's mouth.

- **Evidence of ongoing wear occurring on the occlusal splint**
  If you see evidence of ongoing wear occurring in an occlusal splint, then you may need to consider long-term splint therapy for that patient - especially if they are very heavily bruxist. You need to warn the patient regarding potential chipping or breakage of new restorations in future.

- **The need for further exploratory laboratory procedures**
  When a patient's muscles are very stiff, a lucia jig or leaf gauge might not help in these patients. You need to give them a Michigan splint to help relax their muscles and in turn allow you to mount some new, more accurate CR models when you need to.

Review appointment

As we discussed, in a review appointment you may see a few small marks on the occlusal surface of the splint (if you have marked it during previous appointment).

The photo in ***Figure 25*** suggests the patient is using the splint but also shows you that they don't suffer from a major case of bruxism.

FIGURE 25

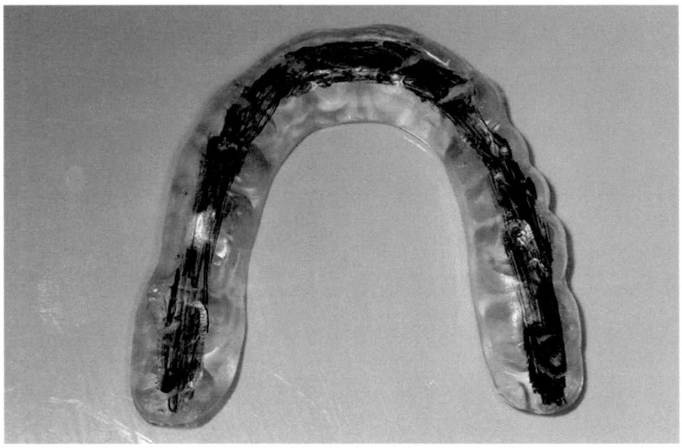

These marks can be removed quite easily, so you need to reassure and give the patient relevant instructions if they are worried about the aesthetics of the splint. However, if they are wearing it at night then aesthetics shouldn't be an issue.

Summary

TMD and parafunctional habits are very important to diagnose and must be dealt with *before* you start any full mouth reconstruction cases. Evidence suggests that occlusal therapy is helpful before and after a full mouth reconstruction or for patients who have TMD diseases.

A carefully made, adjusted and fitted occlusal splint can give a clinician invaluable information with regards to an individual patient, and the feasibility of proposed treatment, by incorporating your restorative height into that occlusal splint.

You should be able to test drive your final occlusal scheme in the patient's mouth, reversibly, without damaging anything. This is one of the safest ways to test your occlusal scheme of the future restorations before you start any comprehensive or full reconstruction cases.

I hope you found this helpful. Now that you have full understanding of occlusion, you are ready to dive deep into treatment planning full mouth reconstruction cases. In the next chapter, we are going to discuss step one of the three-step technique for full mouth reconstruction, which is treatment planning.

If you haven't already done so, make sure to access the free online Practical Guide to FMR Book Course here:

When you use coupon code 'fmrbook' the course will be free for you.

If you are having issues accessing the link by using the QR code, then make sure to contact me at https://drdevangpatel.com/contact/.

CHAPTER 2

Step 1: Treatment Planning

In this chapter we are going to discuss treatment planning for full mouth reconstruction cases.

It's often been said that poor planning leads to poor results. Not laying the groundwork will lead to complications during the later stages of any unplanned treatment. This means you need to write down every single appointment in detail, including your aim for each one.

Of course, not every case will go exactly as you planned and there will always be something that you haven't accounted for.

Yet proper planning will leave you equipped to deal with 90% of whatever you'll come across when doing a full mouth reconstruction case. This is absolutely the key.

Before we discuss treatment planning for full mouth reconstruction cases, we need to understand some of the basic principles of treatment planning which is also helpful in our day to day dentistry.

Fundamentals of treatment planning

There are some basic principles of treatment planning.

Phase 1: Diagnosis and treatment planning phase

Table 2 gives an overview of the diagnosis and treatment planning phase.

Table 2:

GATHER DATA

History: General, Dental, Medial
Radiographic examination
Clinical examination
Other diagnostic aids

General appraisal
Soft tissue and periodontal exam
Oral hygiene and dental exam
Functional and occlusal exam

Arrive at diagnosis
Differential and/or problem list

Develop Treatment Plan/s
Which is a rational sequence based on urgency first and then on efficiency
Which addresses all known problems
Deals with etiologic factors (preventative)
Relates effectively to the patient

Start by **gathering data.**

Take down a **personal history of the patient**, including their dental and medical history, and do both a radiograph and clinical examination.

Other diagnostic tools you can use to do a general appraisal of the patient include a periodontal assessment, a soft tissue assessment, examining the patient's oral hygiene, and doing a functional and occlusal examination. These are the most appropriate ways to collect data.

Next you're going to form **a diagnosis or differential diagnosis** if you're not sure of the exact issues.

Once finished, you're then going to then develop **a treatment plan or plans** based on your diagnosis. Plans consist of a rational sequence of patient-focused actions, based first on urgency and then on efficiency.

You will need to **address any known problems and deal with etiological factors** relating to that particular patient. In short, you are creating a bespoke plan for the patient.

Let us look at these steps in more detail.

Examination

- **Chief complaint**

  When doing any kind of examination, you need to start with the patient's chief complaint.

  Why are they seeing you? As we discussed in the previous chapters, we need to have a very thorough knowledge of how to carry out an assessment, how to communicate with patients, and how to build rapport with each one.

- **Medical history**

  Medical history is very important when it comes to treatment planning for implant or full mouth reconstruction cases.

  By the time a patient comes to see me, they will have filled out a detailed four-page medical history that will signpost any issues.

  For instance, if a patient has a particular medical condition such as a bleeding disorder, it's vital to be aware of that when you're planning an implant so that you act accordingly.

- **Present dental history**

  We need to know a patient's present dental or past dental history. You need to understand if the patient was a **regular or irregular attendee** and what happened in previous visits.

  If the patient has attended your own practice for a long time then study their notes and their previous dentist's notes (if relevant). This means you will have a lot of information about that patient before you even see them.

- **Patient's social history**

  Smoking: When it comes to doing implants, smoking is linked to a lot of issues. Furthermore if you are undertaking direct bonding and your patient is a smoker, then expect some sort of staining. You need to make the patient aware of these issues before starting any treatment.

  Examine a patient's **history with alcohol.**

  Diet: If a patient drinks tea or coffee regularly, then you can expect some staining around the restoration. If a patient has a lot of sugary drinks or sugar in their diet, then you may start getting secondary caries around your restoration. You need to assess this if you're doing a direct build-up and make sure you eliminate those issues before you start doing any treatment.

Occupation: Some occupations will be affected by the treatment, e.g. if you're doing anterior reconstruction and the shape of the teeth are not correct, then we know that the patient may lisp in the beginning for a little while.

If a patient is camera-facing or customer-facing in their working life then you need to warn them that the treatment might temporarily impact their speech.

❖ **Extraoral assessment**

- When carrying out an extraoral examination you need to assess for **Facial Symmetry.** If a patient's face is not symmetrical, you cannot use it as your smile design reference point - something you will need to accommodate.
- You need to assess a patient's **lymph nodes and look for possible swellings**.
- **Assessment of TMJ**, which involves looking for clicking, crepitus pain, deviation when opening, and limited opening of the mouth. Therefore, record how a patient opens their mouth and the muscles of mastication, assessing each and every muscle to make sure there is no tenderness present. If there is, you need to address this before doing a full mouth reconstruction case. Load test using lucia jig or leaf gauge is a very important test when assessing suitability of TMJ/muscles before carrying out full mouth reconstruction.

❖ **Smile line**

At the same time you need to record whether the patient's smile line is high or low. A low smile line is much easier to manage, especially when the patient doesn't have high aesthetic demands.

However, this doesn't mean that the patient won't want the gingival levels corrected. So discuss all options with them.

Something else to be mindful of is that whenever a patient is in the dental chair, they may not be smiling as widely as they usually do because it's not their natural environment.

Therefore, you need to make sure that you take photographs, but also ask each patient to bring in a photograph from outside a dental environment to see how widely they smile.

❖ **Intraoral assessment**

Here you're going to look at the **soft tissue and gingival biotype,** and check the **six point probing depth** for pockets for the full mouth to have a more detailed map of their periodontal health.

❖ **Patient's oral hygiene**

- Check whether the patient uses a **manual or electric toothbrush.**

- **How many times** a patient brushes their teeth in a day.
- **What type of toothpaste** the patient uses.
- Whether they're using **floss** or any **interdental brushes**.
- Whether they use any **mouthwash.**
- It is very important to check all of the above so that you don't get caught out.

I had one patient who kept coming back with a lot of staining on the restorations, for which I could see no apparent explanation. She had forgotten to mention that she was using 0.2% Chlorhexidine four times a day, which turned out to be the cause of the staining.

So having a detailed assessment of what the patient is using helps both sides understand what they're using and why they're using it. If they need to change anything, it will make them understand why they need to change things.

❖ **Hard tissue**

Looking at the hard tissue will mean checking for **caries,** seeing whether there's any **large or defective restorations**, and whether or not there is an **open margin with direct or indirect restorations** you might need to assess and record.

❖ **Occlusion**

- You need to assess the **occlusal stability, skeletal classification and angle classification** for molars and canines on both the right and left-hand sides.
  Having said that, it's not going to make much difference to your full mouth reconstruction per se, beyond helping you communicate with the laboratory or specialist if you're doing any orthodontic treatment.
- You need to assess the **guidance,** as we discussed during our occlusal examination.
- Record the **CO**, using your leaf gauge to assess the first point of contact.
- Record **the shim stock holds.**
- If there are any **signs of parafunction** then again record them, such as wear facets or indentations on the tongue and cheek areas.
- Record **TSL** (tooth surface loss).
- Record **teeth mobility** or any other findings.

Use the QR code below to download my ebook entitled Comprehensive Guide to Clinical Assessment. It is free for you to download:

Signs and symptoms of parafunction

The main signs and symptoms of parafunction are listed below.

- **TMJ**
  As we discussed previously, record any TMJ symptoms when patients come in with **pain or limited irregular movements.**

- **Muscles**
  Check if a patient has **muscle pain or is experiencing spasms.**

- **Teeth**
  Check for **wear facets, drifting, fracture pain or hypersensitivity.**

- **Restorations**
  See if the patient's fillings have signs of wear, fracture and decementation.

If you see these symptoms, make sure that you get to the bottom of the issues before you do any full mouth reconstruction.

You need to understand why a patient might be having those issues, and once you rectify them you need to tell the patient that those issues can come back again.

Even after you've done a full mouth reconstruction, it doesn't guarantee that a patient won't brux their teeth. Because of that, they might end up breaking their newly-restored teeth.

You are unlikely to be able to control whether this happens. Therefore, it's a risk the patient will have to accept.

Special tests

There are lots of special tests you can do to help you reach the right diagnosis.

- **Transillumination tests**
  You can do **transillumination tests** to see the crack lines.

- **Vitality tests**
  You can do a **vitality test,** whether it be hot, cold or electric. We know that the cold test is not really reliable on its own, so ideally you need to do two tests to find out whether the tooth is vital or not.

- **Percussion tests**
  You need to do **percussion tests** by tapping on vertical and lateral aspects of the tooth. This is because sometimes when you tap vertically, patients might not be in pain. However, they will feel pain on tapping laterally if there is an infection in the periapical area but it is situated lateral to the root.

- **Tooth slooth**
  A tooth slooth is a really good tool to have when you're assessing any cracked teeth. It is a plastic spatula-type instrument with the area raised at the end, which you put in one of the cusps before asking the patient to bite. The idea is to check individual cusps to see if the patient experiences pain with any of them.

- **Radiographs**
  The radiographs we have at our disposal can be used in the form of bitewings, periapicals, occlusal radiographs or CBCT scans.

- **Accurate diagnostic models**
  Accurate diagnostic models are also very helpful in assessing the slide outside a patient's mouth. Many times, when a patient has a slide from CO to ICP, they will have some traumatic damage to the anterior teeth because they're sliding quite rapidly under the forward teeth onto the anterior teeth.

Therefore, if a patient breaks their incisal fillings all the time, it helps in assessing whether or not they have a slide, as this may be the cause of the fracturing of the anterior restoration. It also helps when you are mounting models using an articulator.

- **Diagnostic wax up**
  Sometimes you don't know by just looking at a patient's teeth that you will be able to give patients a smile design that they want. Because of that you may need to do a diagnostic wax up before you come to a conclusion.

  Other times a wax up could be crucial in assessing whether you will be able to do a direct reconstruction or if a patient may need indirect restorations. I use the 2mm rule, **if the thickness of wax is 2mm or more then I would consider that tooth for an indirect restoration.**

- **Photographs**
  If you take photographs with really good resolution and magnify them, you will be able to assess things more effectively than just with your normal eyesight.

- **Selective anesthesia**
  If a patient comes in with pain and you can't locate whether it's in the upper or lower jaw, you can anesthetise one jaw and see if the patient is still in pain. If the patient is not in pain in the area where you gave the local anesthetic, then you've located which jaw the pain is coming from.

  Numbing an individual tooth is a bit trickier as it's not really accurate, but if your patient is not sure because they have a referred pain from one jaw to the other, then this technique works really well.

- **Test cavity**
  A test cavity can be done when you're not sure whether a patient's tooth is vital or non-vital. In this technique you refrain from giving a patient local anesthetic and then start drilling the tooth as if you are going to do a root canal treatment. If the patient feels pain, that means the tooth is vital.

  Having said that, there have been many incidents where dentists have drilled through to the pulp on a vital tooth because of the cold water generating less heat, which means the patient doesn't have a chance to experience any pain before the pulp chamber has a perforation.

So overall, a test cavity is an unreliable method for checking whether a patient is in pain or whether a tooth is vital or not.

Tooth by tooth prognosis

In full mouth reconstruction cases I always make a note of each individual tooth, assessing what type of restoration that tooth has and if there is any available dentin for me to restore the tooth (***Table 3***).

Table 3:

Tooth	Type of restoration/ surface involved	Availability of dentin sufficient/ moderate/ insufficient (TRI)	TTP	Mobility	Vitality (Endo Ice)	Vitality (EPT)	Other comments (radiographs)
18							
17							
16							
15							
14							
…							

I also check to see if it is heavily filled, whether there is pain on the percussion, whether the tooth has mobility, what its vital status is and if there are any specific comments I want to make about it, such as a post and core crown or marginal caries around the crown which you can see in the radiographs of periapical lesion.

If you are getting overwhelmed by the treatment planning, then this is the best way to break things down to a tooth-by-tooth prognosis, which in turn breaks down treatment in a manageable way.

Phase 2: Stabilisation/disease control phase:

The next stage is stabilisation phase, where you're going to extract the teeth which need to come out and give the patient a provisional restoration if they want one.

If it's a posterior tooth and the patient is happy to leave the gap for a while, then leave the gap.

You can do a periodontal assessment and treatment by giving the patient a six-point pocket charting, a full mouth cleaning, and a referral if necessary to a specialist.

If a patient has experienced inadequate endodontic treatment and if you're going to change or restore a tooth with the crown, the tooth should be retreated before the crown is done. I always tell the patient that I understand that the tooth is not painful right now, but the root canal treatment is not optimum. By doing a crown on that tooth, we are changing the environment of the tooth. Therefore, it is likely that that tooth will get painful or symptomatic. The patient may need a re-root canal treatment, which will be a shame after doing the new crown. Because of that I would recommend that the patient redoes the root canal treatment if it's not optimum.

Obviously make sure that before that treatment a core investigation is done, building those teeth up with composite if you need to. Control the cause of the disease by doing a diet chart and a case analysis, and make sure you've done the periodontal assessment and risk assessment before you start the treatment.

Phase 3: Definitive/restorative phase:

Once you've done the stabilisation phase and assessed all those issues, you're now coming into the definitive restorative phase.

You will need to do another consultation, including doing a further assessment of smile design and a diagnostic wax up before finalising the treatment plan and considering whether the patient needs orthodontic treatment or whitening.

Furthermore, you will need to consider what type of restoration you are going to do (direct, indirect or a combination restoration), including maybe an anterior direct buildup, a posterior indirect restoration, or whether you'll go with a conformative or reorganised approach as we discussed before.

So all this will be assessed in a definitive phase; if you're doing a direct build-up, decide which technique you are going to do. Are you going to do a freehand build-up? Are you going to use clear indices?

If you're doing indirect restorations, are you going to do crowns, using different materials?Are you going to do onlays or veneers? You need to consider this while you're doing treatment planning because the patient's estimate or fees will depend on this.

By this point, because you will have investigated all the teeth you will be able to give patients a much better idea about the treatment plan, along with realistic fees related to that treatment plan.

You also need to decide whether the patient needs crown-lengthening, depending on their gingival level, or if the patient needs fixed, removal or a combination of treatment to replace their missing teeth. If you are giving them something fixed, are you going to do implants or fixed bridges for such patients?

Once you've done that, you are then going to do anterior reconstruction, which once completed will mean you need to decide how you're going to stabilise the posterior teeth by doing the provisional restoration using the wax up or doing GIC stops. You will possibly need to take new impressions once you build the anterior teeth to wax up the posterior teeth again, so that you can use the index technique followed by posterior build up. We will discuss this in detail in Chapters 3 which deals with anterior reconstruction and Chapter 4 in which we will discuss posterior reconstruction.

Phase 4: Maintenance phase

Once you finish everything you will put the patient into a maintenance phase, where you're going to give them a Michigan splint to maintain your restoration. You can give patients a soft mouth guard or a clear retainer (like an Essix retainer or Dual arch B splint) if they have had orthodontic treatment.

However, a soft mouth guard is not ideal for TMJ issues or patients with bruxism, so my choice would be a Michigan splint or Essix retainer or dual arch B splint if a patient has had braces.

Regular visits to the hygienist are needed. You need to emphasise to the patient that just because they have had all this treatment done, it doesn't mean that they can disappear and never come back.

You also need to put the patient on high fluoride toothpaste, especially if they have a high caries risk.

Additional maintenance of your direct restorations will be needed by doing polishing, repairing chips if needed and assessing the implant prosthesis.

Above all, you need to make the patient understand what is involved in doing a full mouth reconstruction case. Sometimes I walk them through this whole scenario from the first phase to the last phase and explain everything in detail to them. This increases their sense of value, making the patient understand why they are paying so much - which is basically because it requires so much work!

To sum up...

Overall, you need to ask yourself one fundamental question: 'will this patient's oral health be better off when I have finished with the treatment?'

Factors affecting in general treatment planning

There are certain factors (***Table 4***) which can affect treatment planning, related to **patients, dentists or other things in general**.

Table 4:

Patient Factors	**Dentist Factors**
Patient's preferences	Dentist's knowledge
Motivation	Experience and Training
Systemic Health	Laboratory Support
Emotional Status	Dentist-patient compatibility
Financial Stability	Availability of specialists
	Functional, aesthetic and technical demands
General	
Pulpal and periapical diagnosis	
Periodontal condition	
Restorability of the the teeth	
Individual tooth prognosis	
Prognosis of key teeth	

- **The patient factor**
  It could be that the patient just prefers a certain type of treatment. It will be your job to advise them on their preference and whether you feel comfortable doing that treatment or not.

If a 20-year-old patient comes to me with crowding issues and asks me to give them veneers because it's a quick fix, I will refuse to do that treatment. This is because I know that it's unlikely to be in that patient's best interests.

You also need to gauge whether a **patient is motivated enough,** especially when you're doing a case of full mouth reconstruction. This does not work in the same way as putting in a single filling, where you just do the job and then the patient leaves.

Full mouth reconstruction involves many appointments and a lot of effort from both you and the patient. A sense of enthusiasm is of the utmost importance to see you both through.

On top of this, you need to understand the **patient's systemic health** and whether they can physically cope with the treatment.

The emotional status of the patient is also very important. If the patient is not emotionally stable, I will not treat them.

Unfortunately, patients can make decisions without properly thinking them through. If they have made the decision while in a poor mental state, then once you finish the treatment you risk the patient coming to you and claiming that this was not what they wanted, blaming it on a lack of communication.

In extreme cases this can then lead to dento-legal issues. Therefore, only proceed if you are sure that the patient is mentally prepared.

Lastly, you will need to assess the **patient's financial capability,** as unfortunately there will always be patients who need the treatment but cannot afford the ideal option. In this case you and the patient both need to come to an appropriate compromise which is suitable for both of you.

- **The dentist factor**

When it comes to the dentist factor, **dental knowledge** is really important. After all, it's the reason you are reading this book, so that you can improve your knowledge in order to take on more complex cases.

Experience and training also helps, as if you are more experienced and have undertaken more treatments then that will boost your confidence.

Whenever you're doing indirect restorations, **laboratory support** is a must. Many dentists have been let down on this front, as it's possible to control a lot of things clinically but not in the lab. If the technicians are not producing high quality work then you cannot expect to have an excellent final result.

You also need to ensure that you and the patient are **compatible.** In other words, you both need to like each other! If you don't, then there is no point in going forward as it will be challenging seeing each other a lot.

If you don't do a certain type of treatment - let's say orthodontic or surgical treatment - then you need to have a **network of specialists** around you that can provide support when you need it.

And finally, you need to understand a **patient's functional, aesthetic and the restorative demands** in cases of full mouth reconstruction.

- **The general factor**
  Common general factors include **pulpal and periapical diagnosis, the patient's periodontal condition, and the restorability of the teeth.**

  I often tell patients that unless I remove all the old fillings from the teeth, I will not know whether a tooth needs a crown, needs to come out or whether a simple filling will do. I also tell patients that removing an existing large restoration or a crown may mean a tooth can become symptomatic, leading to them possibly needing a root canal in that tooth.

  It's therefore better to be upfront in explaining any risks before you start the treatment. After you start the treatment, any problem that comes up which wasn't discussed will sound like an excuse.

  You then need to decide on the **prognosis of individual teeth and the prognosis of key teeth,** especially the posterior most tooth in the arch if you're doing a removable prosthesis case.

- **The individual factor**
  Let's look at some of the individual factors which can affect your treatment planning.

  - **Orthodontics: forgotten discipline for adults needing FMR**
    Orthodontics are often an overlooked treatment for adult full mouth reconstruction cases. Although it's now becoming more popular for cosmetic reasons, it's not that popular when it comes to doing full mouth reconstructions.

Yet it is a vital tool for dentists who are doing such complex work. I would urge you to get to grips with the principle of orthodontics and what they can help you achieve.

- **Crowns and extracoronal restorations: things to consider when planning treatment**
  Whenever I'm doing crowns or extracoronal restorations, I always ask myself whether it will last 10 years or more. In dentistry 10 years is a golden number, with anything above that considered arguably to be a success.

You therefore need to discuss this with each patient, as you don't want to give them the illusion that whatever they have in their mouth is going to last them for a lifetime.

Of course, our aim would be to make it last for as long as possible; but as long as they understand that 10 years or above is considered to be a success, then they will have a more realistic perspective regarding the treatment plan.

Now planning for the treatment involves analysing three aspects:

1) **THE PATIENT**: I'm looking to see if the patient's expectations are realistic. Will they be able to tolerate the treatment and then maintain the restorations? Some patients can't sit in the chair for long enough, while others won't be able to keep their mouths open wide for long enough. I'm similarly always assessing whether or not my skills as a dentist are good enough to provide high-quality restorations. Can I justify the changes I'm going to make in a patient's mouth by ensuring they receive the desired outcome? You always need to justify whether what you're doing to a patient is worth it.

2) **MOUTH AND TEETH:** Secondly, I'm looking at the mouth and teeth. Can the patient and I both control the oral environment to minimise the risk of disease or damage in the long term?

   We both need to work together, which includes the patient's plaque control being good enough, managing their overall oral hygiene better, and addressing the risk of the caries in the future.

   We need to discuss the treatment and make sure that the patient understands that teeth can still get decayed, even though they have crowns, onlays or restorations.

   Furthermore, has the risk of damage from occlusion been minimised? As dentists it's our job to make sure the occlusion does not damage a patient's new restorations.

3) **THE TOOTH:** are the foundations of the teeth biologically and biomechanically sound? Does the patient have any periodontal issues? Are their teeth endodontically sound, and has there been endodontic treatment?

   We've all seen a lot of post and core restorations with no endodontic treatment or very short root canal treatments and no periapical pathology. If you're doing full mouth reconstruction cases and you need to change a crown, you need to make a decision about whether you're going to just ignore the root canal-treated tooth or you're going to remove the treatment and do a new post and core crown - or if in extreme cases, you're going to extract that tooth.

   Extracting such a tooth and placing an implant can be considered in some cases, as you cannot be certain whether the patient is going to have any issues in the future once you've re-done the post and core crowns.

   You will need to check whether the tooth itself is strong enough to withstand your preparation of the crown, and whether the preparation will be retentive enough if you're doing a conventional restoration.

   Can you isolate that tooth with a rubber dam if you're doing an adhesive technique, or do you want to do a deep marginal elevation in order to isolate the tooth you'll need to put the rubber dam on the tooth?

   Finally, is there enough space for you to restore the tooth? Having said that, this is not really an issue because when you're doing a full mouth reconstruction you are almost certainly raising OVD, which means you're going to get a little bit of extra space to help you in doing restorations.

Endodontics vs implants

The other question you need to ask is whether to save the tooth by doing endodontic treatment or go for extraction instead.

Which decision you make will come down to three factors:

1) **Patient-related factors** – These include systemic or oral health, comfort and treatment perceptions. If the patient has an intense bleeding disorder, then there is a high likelihood that they will not be able to have an implant. If that is the case, then I'll try and do anything to save that tooth, even if it means heroic treatment. Because if that

tooth comes out then the patient may not be able to have the implant. The worst case scenario is that if it comes out they can always have a fixed bridge done or a denture. However, try to keep the tooth as long as you can.

2) **Tooth and periodontium related factors** - So if the tooth is grade 3 mobile, then there's no point in keeping that tooth. If a patient has an endodontic lesion and you feel that the tooth is otherwise sound, then it's better to try and do a root canal and get rid of that lesion. If there's a dark discoloured tooth, then root canal treatment, internal whitening and a crown usually sorts the problem out.

3) **The quality of the bone** - If I've done a CT scan and therefore know the patient doesn't have enough bone and will need an extreme bone grafting if they lose that tooth, then I'll try and do all I can to save that tooth.

These are the three factors you really need to understand when you are debating whether to do endodontic treatment or an implant. However, I have a very simple approach to treatment: if I can save the tooth I will always try and save the tooth.

The only thing I do not recommend is doing apicoectomies because they can ruin the area which may need future implant. It may allow the patient to keep that tooth for some time, but when it comes to doing implants later on the patient will have a lot of scar tissue, which can jeopardise future treatment.

Periodontal condition: maintain or extract?

With periodontal conditions, you need to ask the question of whether you are going to keep a tooth which has a grade one to two mobility, or you're going to have it out. Otherwise, you may get continued bone loss, with the patient having severe bone loss after two or three years later.

It's a quite difficult dilemma, and unfortunately studies rarely help. A study done by McGuire and Nun shows that predicting how long these teeth will last is anyone's guess.

You cannot really predict how long the predominantly affected teeth will last unless they have symptoms such as worsening probing depth, furcation involvement, mobility, and a high percentage of bone loss or a parafunctional habit.

If the patient has all those things and they are getting progressively worse, then maybe you can assume that the tooth will have to come out soon.

Yet in my clinical opinion I've seen patients with grade three mobility in their teeth last those teeth for four or five years, which is why it is very difficult for us to predict that the tooth will have to be extracted.

If you would still feel compelled to make a prediction, then we know from a study by Lang et al that bleeding on probing is a very good indicator of disease progression, and we know that the tooth is getting worse and worse day by day.

This might make your decision a little bit easier, since if the patient still has some bleeding on probing and deep pocketing after treatment, then that means the tooth might have to come out.

However, you still need to understand the other factors. I won't extract teeth which have maybe 2mm or 3mm of pocketing and bleeding on probing. Conversely, if a patient has 9mm or 10mm of pocketing and there's bleeding on probing, then those teeth will have to come out.

Even though it's not the most reliable factor, bleeding on probing is one of the most important factors when it comes to assessing a tooth and its periodontal condition.

2.1 Treatment Planning in Full Mouth Reconstruction

Before we press on, let's look at the simplified steps involved in full mouth reconstruction. Remember, this workflow is for adhesive DIRECT full mouth reconstruction.

Step 1: Treatment planning

So you start with a comprehensive assessment, an impression, with the interocclusal records to get models mounted in ICP, CR, or CO depending on your treatment planning. You will also need a diagnostic wax up and trial of that wax up, such as a mock-up in the patient's mouth.

Step 2: Anterior buildups

Once you've done all this, you can then do upper and lower anterior (canine to canine) buildups.

The protocol I follow is to do treatment planning and then an anterior buildup using upper and lower anterior definitive wax up and stents and posterior temporaries using a wax up or GIC stops.

Step 3: Posterior buildups

Once I've done an anterior reconstruction I will move on to a posterior construction with a definitive restoration either one arch at a time - (lower arch first and then upper arch) or one side at a time (you can choose any side right or left to do first). That will depend on whether cosmetically or aesthetically you or your technician can maintain the arch and keep the occlusal plane flat.

If you both can, then I personally prefer the lower posterior first followed by the upper posteriors.

Once you have finished the treatment, you need to protect your restoration by giving the patient some sort of occlusal appliance such as Michigan splint and a maintenance regime.

In this part we will discuss Step 1 which is treatment planning aspect of full mouth reconstruction which is the most important aspect.

We have already discussed the fundamentals of basic treatment planning. Now let's discuss things you need to consider for planning full mouth reconstruction cases.

Planning by asking questions

Treatment planning involves various decision-making steps Let's look at some of the criteria to help your decision-making during treatment planning easier.

1. A conformative or reorganised approach?

One of the most important questions to ask is whether you're going to approach this treatment as conformative or reorganised.

- During many restorative procedures a decision may need to be made about whether to work with an existing occlusal scheme or modify it for a specific purpose.
- In most instances such as single tooth restorations, the overall occlusal scheme will remain unchanged after a restoration. This is called a conformative approach.
- When an occlusal relationship needs to be altered as part of a treatment, it is often called a reorganised approach. Most full mouth reconstruction cases will fall into this category. You might not increase OVD, but because you're changing so many occlusal surfaces, by definition you will be doing a reorganised approach.

Conformative approach

Indications:

- Single unit.
- Symptom-free patient, the teeth to be restored are bounded, a good stable occlusion, stable stops and ICP.
- Large horizontal-small vertical slide.
- Patient with a previous TMJ problem.
- Re-restoration of anterior teeth with stable posterior teeth.
- With a re-restoration of the anterior teeth, if the rest of the mouth is stable and if you're just doing anterior crowns (maybe six), then you can still do a conformative approach.

When it comes to such an approach, we have the following advantages:

- No adaptation, or very little, of the patient's neuromuscular system.
- Treatment is confined to the restored tooth.
- Index technique can be used.
- Treatment is confined to the restored tooth, so you can use the index technique if a patient comes to you with good anatomy of the teeth, just taking the indices of the teeth and creating a new restoration with the same anatomy.
- If you have a small number of restorations, then the lab process will be easy.
- However, when you're doing a full mouth reconstruction, you're probably doing a restoration for every single tooth but also reorganising the occlusion.

Reorganised approach

The advantages of a reorganised approach are:

- Preparation of teeth does not result in unwanted change of jaw relationship as new CR position is used to restore all the teeth.
- Greater control over the future relationship of the teeth.
- Stable occlusion, in harmony with border movements.
- Iatrogenic deflective contacts are not introduced as the occlusal scheme is changed.
- Control over interocclusal contacts.
- Posterior stability.

How to choose between the conformative and the reorganised approach?

So how do you choose what kind of approach you're going to use - conformative or reorganised? Before you make a decision, you should consider the following:

- The length of the slide makes a difference. If the patient has got a large horizontal and small vertical slide then you may not want to do full mouth reconstruction. Unless you are very experienced, and you may want to conform to the patient's original occlusion and try to minimise the number of restorations you'll do.
- When you have supraeruption of the teeth and you cannot really change this discrepancy. In that case, you may want to conform or remove those discrepancies, by extracting the teeth or through orthodontic treatment, before you do any full mouth reconstruction.
- The patient's ability to tolerate a new bite is really important, so if the patient comes in with any stiff joints or pain you need to possibly give them a Michigan splint first before you go ahead with full mouth reconstruction.

This is because the Michigan splint will help you understand if the patient can tolerate a raised OVD.

2. Are the teeth in the right place?

Whether you need to move the gums, the teeth or both is something really important to consider when assessing a patient's orthodontic status.

With this patient in ***Figure 26a*** and ***Figure 26b*** you can see that the teeth and gums are not in the right position. The patient certainly needs orthodontic treatment followed by a possible crown-lengthening. If the orthodontic treatment hasn't solved that, then it will most likely be a full mouth reconstruction case.

FIGURE 26a

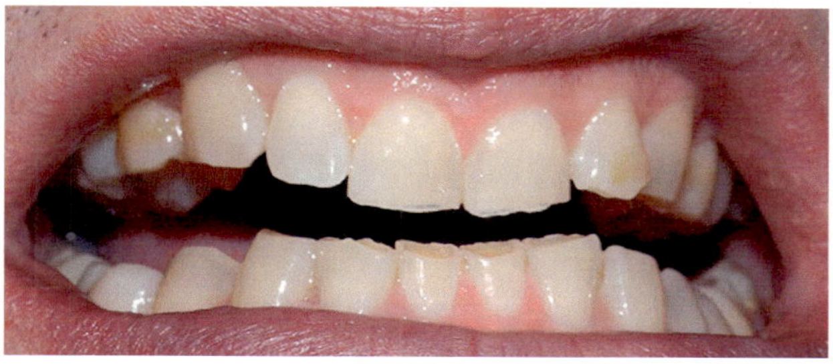

FIGURE 26b

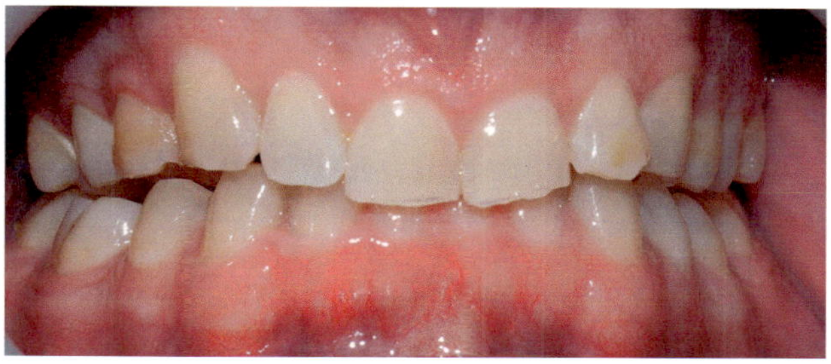

Therefore, if you start doing full month reconstruction for this patient, all you're going to do is incorporate the same issue that was in your restoration, as you haven't changed the position of the patient's teeth.

3. Patient-based factors

- **Assess the patient**

Can you both get on with each other?

You need to make sure that you like working with each other. If you don't like the patient or the patient doesn't like you, then there is no point doing a full mouth reconstruction for that patient. It's a harsh reality but an important decision as you are going to see each other a lot if you proceed.

Furthermore, since you're going to do treatment for their whole mouth you will be responsible for their oral health for years to come. If you don't get on with each other, then it is important to tell the patient that it's in their best interests to find someone else.

Can you fulfill the patient's goals?

So maybe you get on with each other but the patient has really unrealistic goals which mean you cannot give them what they want. This might be the best time to say to a patient that they should seek a second opinion.

Non-compliance from the patient (do they value what you're doing?)

Many times, patients have reasonable expectations but won't comply with your instructions. So if you ask them to do something and they don't do it - such as not cleaning their teeth properly - then you may choose not to treat. Your treatment may fail because of their ignorance, because they are busy, or because their lifestyle is such that they cannot take care of their teeth properly.

This needs to be fully assessed beforehand.

4. Condition of TMJ

It's worth considering the condition of TMJ. As we discussed, during an occlusal examination if I've done the load test and the patient is in pain with TMJ or muscles, then that patient is getting a Michigan splint until there is no pain during the load test. I will not proceed with full mouth reconstruction if a patient is still in pain.

If the patient is not in pain with TMJ during the load test, and I can manipulate that jaw nicely, then I'll go ahead with the full mouth reconstruction without giving them any occlusal appliance.

If the patient is not in pain with TMJ but I cannot manipulate the jaw properly, then I am going to give them a Michigan splint to relax their muscles so I can get a more accurate CR position. However, you can use Kois deprogrammer if you prefer.

Sometimes a patient cannot locate their bite properly. In this case also, I would prefer to give them a Michigan splint to relax their jaw, or any sort of deprogrammer (as we discussed earlier) to have the same effect before I record that CR position.

These are my two go-to deprogrammers when it comes to recording a patient's CR (See ***Figure 27a, lucia jig*** and ***27b, Huffman's leaf gauge***).

FIGURE 27a

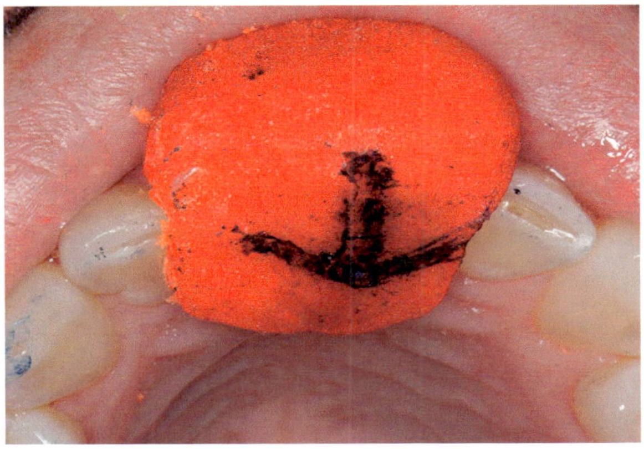

FIGURE 27b

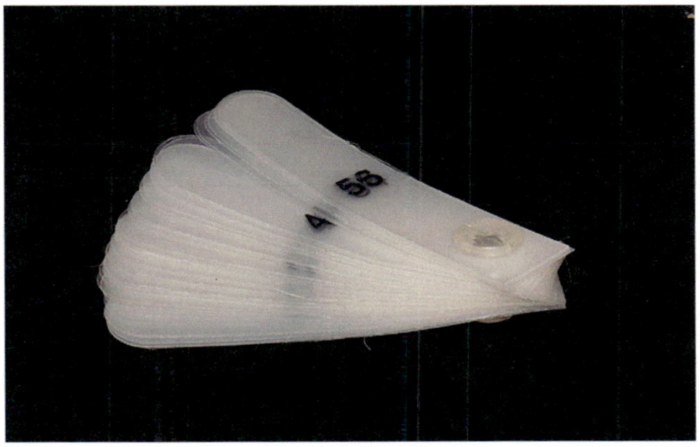

5. What type of wear?

Another question to ask is what type of wear the patient has.

❖ **Pattern/extent of teeth wear**

This is very important. I tend to ask patients to move their upper and lower jaw in a specific direction so that their wear facets meet each other. Then I can see where that jaw is going while they're grinding their teeth, especially for those patients with attrition cases because of bruxism.

You need to make sure when you're doing a final restoration that you haven't created interference when they grind their teeth. If you have made a custom guidance table replicating all the jaw movements, then you may be able to replicate that in the patient's mouth.

- It's important to gauge whether the wear is generalised or localised. If a patient only has anterior wear and no wear with the posterior teeth, then you'll be considering DAHL treatment.
- If the patient has anterior or posterior wear, then you can also consider orthodontic treatment to move the teeth and create space for your restoration.
- Assess how many teeth have wear. This also helps you decide whether you're going to have a reorganised or conformative approach. If a patient has generalised wear then you're going to have a reorganised approach.

- However, if a patient has got wear in only one tooth then doing a reorganised approach will be too invasive.
- Determine the upper incisor length on show while at rest and smiling and that will help you in assessing whether to increase the OVD or do crown-lengthening.

So if patients showing a full central incisor (full width and length) on smile and have wear, then that means there is a dental alveolar compensation. They haven't actually lost OVD; therefore if you increase OVD you're going to give them big long teeth.

So in this case you may need to avoid or minimise the increase of OVD, or do a restoration with crown-lengthening or orthodontic treatment, moving those teeth back into that position. ***Figure 28a*** and ***FIgure 28b*** shows a patient with intact anterior teeth and the same patient in ***Figure 29a*** and ***29b*** showing severe localised posterior wear.

FIGURE 28a

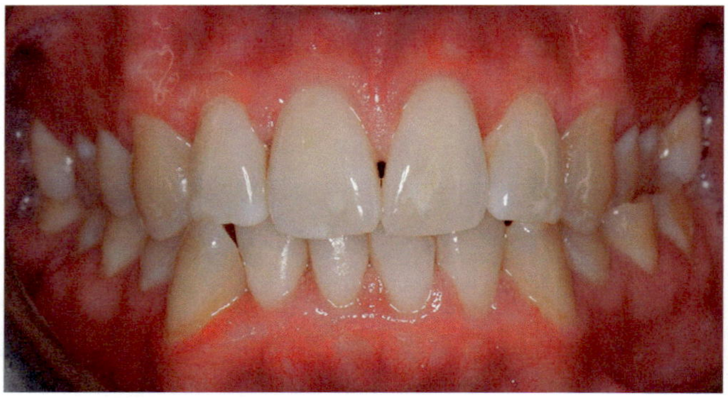

FIGURE 28b

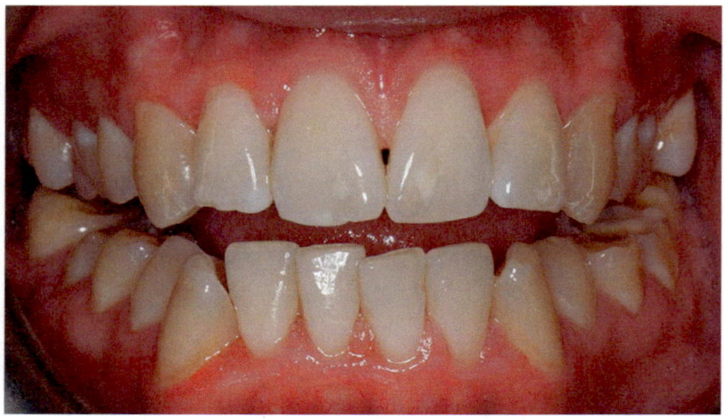

FIGURE 29a

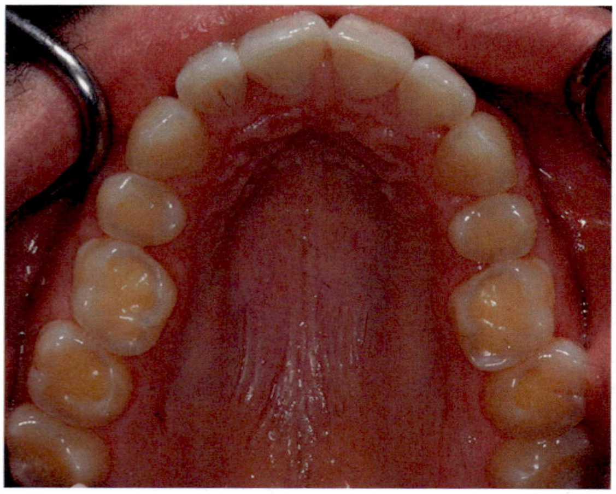

FIGURE 29b

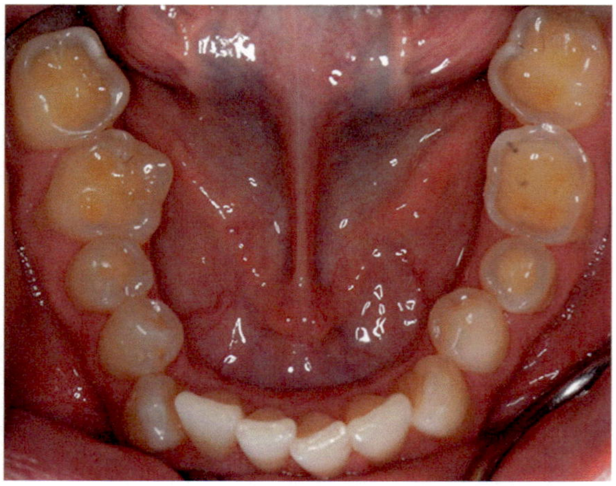

In ***Figure 30a, 30b*** and ***30c*** what we've done is build the posterior teeth first. This is because when you do orthodontic treatment first, you often cannot guarantee that you're going to get the space you require.

I therefore tend to build the posterior teeth first and then do orthodontic treatment to bring the teeth together. This is only relevant for localised posterior wear. For localised anterior wear, we would carry out DAHL or consider orthodontic treatment.

Of course, this is risky and that's why I don't do indirect restoration. As a result, these teeth were built using direct restoration. This provides some flexibility in adjusting those restorations by reducing or adding resin if I need to.

FIGURE 30a

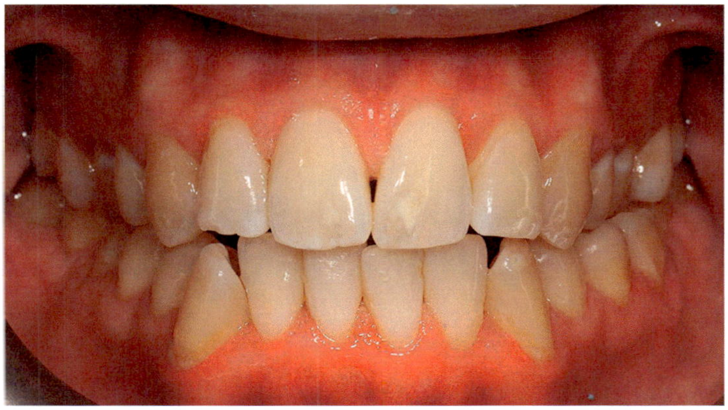

FIGURE 30b

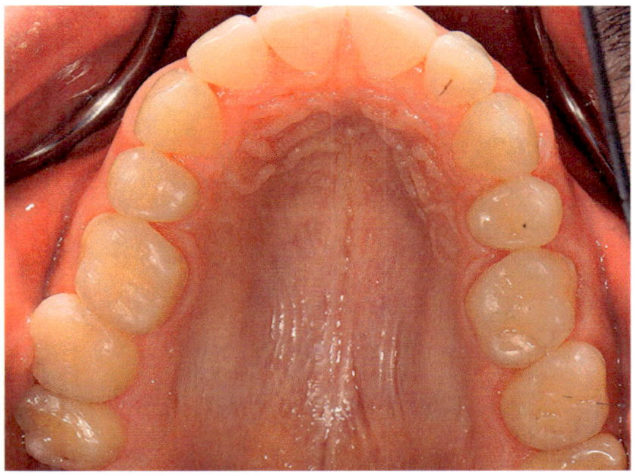

FIGURE 30c

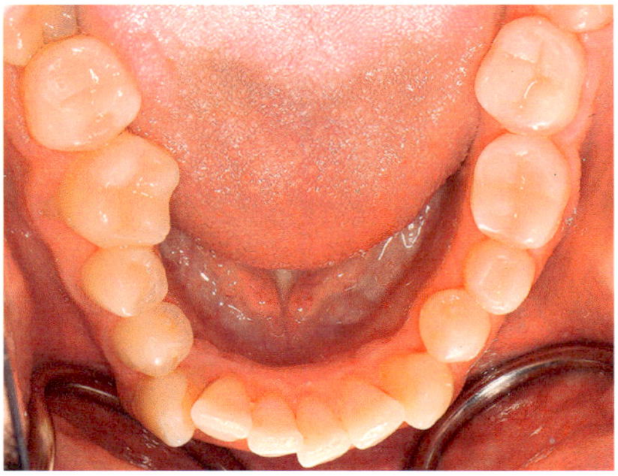

Once I'm finished with the orthodontic treatment, if I wish I can then convert to an indirect restoration if that's what is needed.

6. Occlusal plane

Something else to consider is the occlusal plane is the **Curve of Spee.**

The Curve of Spee to needs to be as flat as possible. This is an important factor when deciding if single arch or a dual arch reconstruction is needed.

When you are doing your planning, it makes a difference if the occlusal plane, especially on the lower arch, is flat. If the lower arch is flat, then most likely the upper arch would be flat as well if they are all in contact.

It will also help you in deciding whether you're going to DAHL those anterior teeth or not or whether the patient is going to need orthodontic treatment.

If the occlusal plane is raised anteriorly, that means there is a dental alveolar compensation, and just putting some composite on there will not allow you to move the teeth back to their normal position.

That's why you may need orthodontic treatment first before you build up the restoration.

It can also help you decide how much opening you need to do, because once again, if you're adding a lot of material on the anterior and not looking at the occlusal plane, you might get an uneven occlusal plane.

Why is this so important?

As we discussed in our first chapter, if the Curve of Spee is steep then anterior guidance will have to be steeper, to disengage the posterior teeth.

Because the anterior guidance will be steeper, the patient will have a restricted envelope of function and will feel that their jaw is locked in. They will grind more, affecting that envelope of function. That's why we want shallow guidance and a flatter Curve of Spee.

If you ignore the patient's midline on ***Figure 31a*** and look at the lower arch, which is flat, then you'll see that is the easier case to manage. In ***Figure 31b,*** you'll see that the patient has a slightly uneven Curve of Spee, but now if I only restore the anterior teeth, then the curve will be exaggerated.

FIGURE 31a

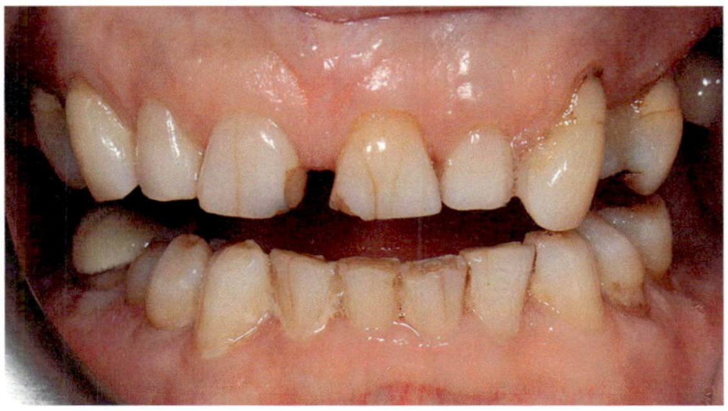

FIGURE 31b

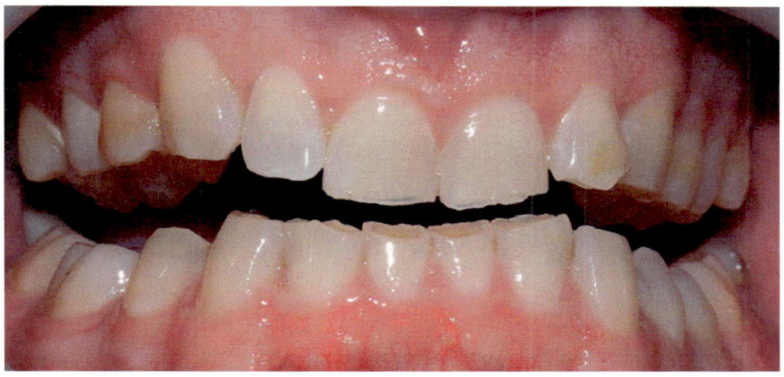

7. Limiting factors

So what are the limiting factors when you are discussing or planning treatments?

- One factor is a **newly-fitted crown** which a patient may not want to change.
  There are a number of patients who have come to see me for an implant or full mouth reconstruction for whom another dentist has just done some treatment, such as a newly fitted crown. Now that I'm doing full mouth reconstruction, where I'm raising their bite, by default I need to change all the restorations in their mouth.

  They may not want to have this newly-fitted, expensive crown removed. I might not want to remove it either if I know the crown is sound. In these cases, it becomes a little bit difficult to justify taking that crown out. You may want to then try and see if you can fit your treatment within the specified dimensions.

- If the patient has a **post** and **core crown** with poorly root canal-treated teeth, then again it becomes a dilemma about whether you're going to keep it. If so, are you just changing the crown, changing the post and core as well, or are you going to redo the root canal treatment? There are a lot of decisions to be made here, and they merit careful consideration.

- If a patient has an **existing implant** and doesn't know what the brand or make of the implant is, then it becomes a bit trickier to make new crowns. This is because if you're

increasing their OVD then it is likely that the implant crown or bridge will need to be replaced. Sometimes, even if the restoration looks fine.
That will be an additional cost to the patient, so their financial situation is something you need to consider too.

- Patients may need **orthodontic treatment** first if they have a severely supraerupted tooth. If so you need to really decide whether ortho is appropriate, or if extraction of that tooth is a simpler route or you will accept this and work around it with a compromised result.

Treatment planning

Identifying issues before you start the treatment is really important part of your planning process.

In ***Figure 32a*** and ***Figure 32b*** you can see a patient who requires orthodontic treatment first in order to do a full mouth reconstruction. The patient in ***Figure 32c*** also requires orthodontic treatment.

FIGURE 32a

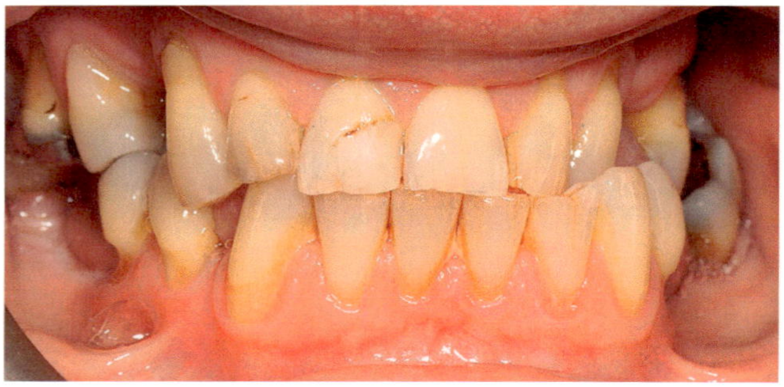

FIGURE 32b

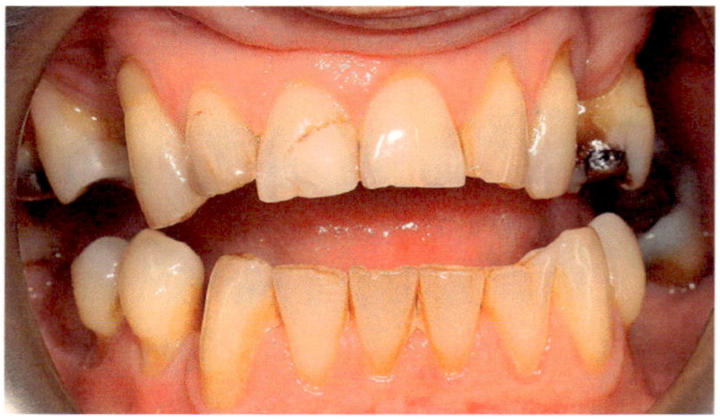

FIGURE 32c

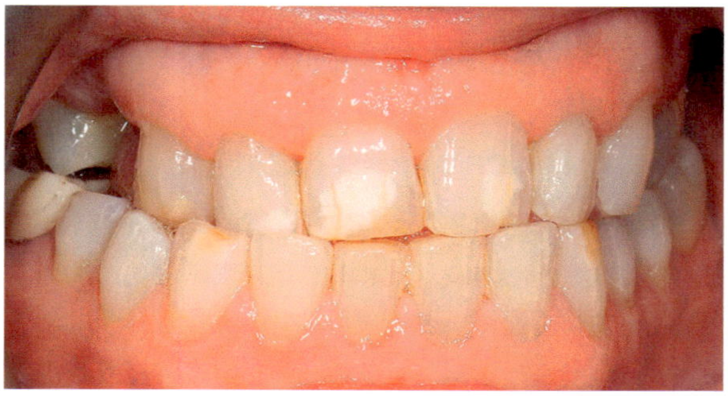

If a patient comes to me with their upper tooth supraerupted into the lower cavity, then the patient needs the orthodontic treatment. The case in ***Figure 33*** is an easier case because you're going to just change the crown on the upper arch and create space for lower restoration.

FIGURE 33

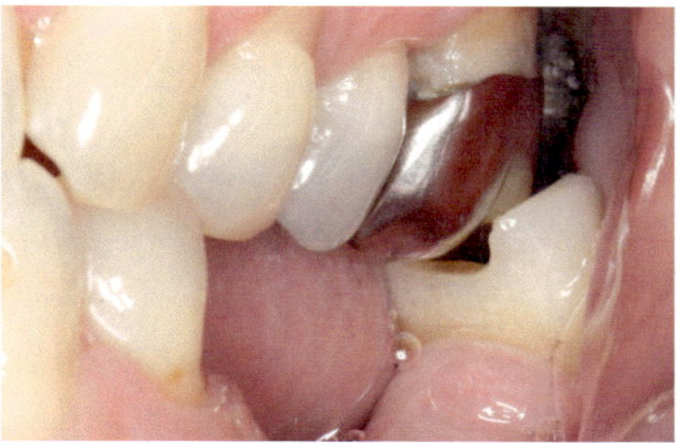

In ***Figure 34a*** and ***34b*** we have a class III bite with an upper left second molar (LL7) that is very supraerupted, to the point where it's almost crossing the lower left first molar. No matter how much of a vertical dimension you raise, you will never get an occlusal plane straight. In that case, you either have to accept that position or extract the UL7 and then decide to replace the teeth.

In this case I accepted the position of the seven because the patient could not afford an implant. We used the UL7 as an anchor tooth for the clasps of denture.

What does this mean? This means there's a compromise in the occlusal scheme, and we need to make the patient understand that this is the compromise treatment. What we're doing is not ideal.

FIGURE 34a

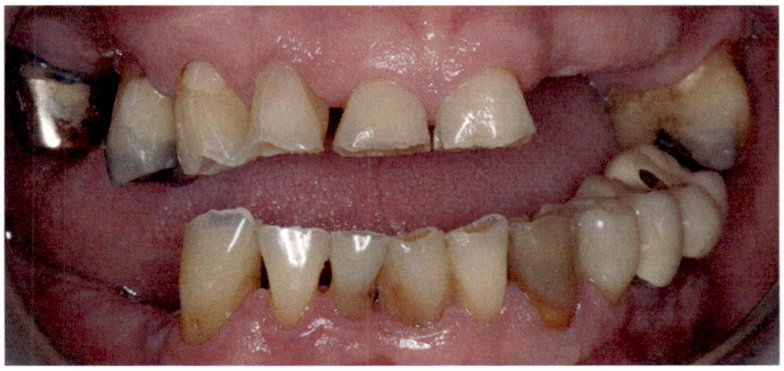

FIGURE 34b

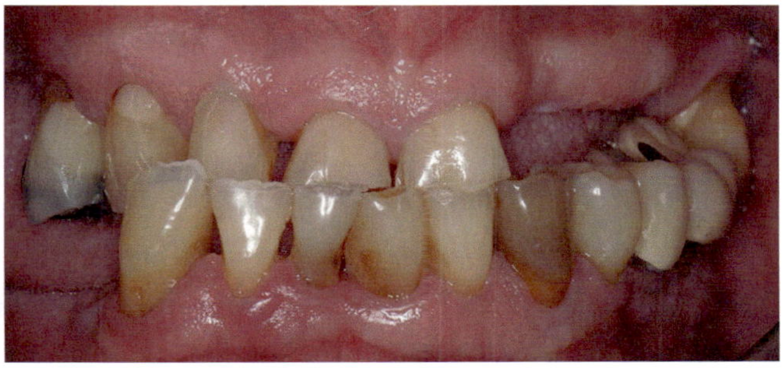

❖ Managing risk

When you are planning a full mouth reconstruction you need to try and manage some key areas of risk.

You need to make sure you assess a patient for **parafunctional habits**. If they are bruxist and grind their teeth then there is a likelihood that they will be doing that on your restorations as well and you need to warn the patient accordingly.

You need to assess if patients are motivated enough. If not, then don't treat them, even if they are willing to pay you. If they're not motivated, then they're not going to take care of what you have done to their mouth, which means they will have issues in future.

If they have a poor sense of oral hygiene, then this needs to be improved first before you start doing a full mouth reconstruction. If a patient is non-compliant, which means not doing what you've asked them to do, then it is highly likely that you will have some issues with your treatment.

Lastly, inform patients about possible complications. Tell them that root canal treatments, implants and restorations can fail in the long run.

For instance, I tell patients that they will break restorations if they are bruxist. We will try and help them control the forces they are applying to the restoration, but they will inevitably apply force to new restorations, breaking or chipping them, and they will have to pay the fees to treat them in future if that happens, depending on the guarantees you have given them, which can be between one and three years. So you can have that structure in place, but the patient needs to be aware that they need to pay for any damage which is caused. I always tell patients that restorations are not for a lifetime. If you do this before the treatment happens, then it is more likely to be a process of informed consent.

If instead you only tell patients this after a complication has happened, then that will almost certainly be considered an excuse. Therefore make sure that you have informed the patient well enough and that you plan things out properly before you progress to full mouth reconstruction.

I hope you found this helpful and that you feel much more confident in the process of planning some of the treatments. In the next chapter we will discuss things you need to consider while raising OVD.

2.2 Increasing OVD

In this chapter, we are going to discuss various aspects related to increasing OVD.

What skills are needed for increasing OVD?

Before we start, I would like to address some of the concerns dentists tend to have. They do not feel that they have enough experience or knowledge to increase OVD.

I firmly believe that if you can provide a patient with a Michigan Splint (***Figure 35a*** and ***Figure 35b***) and take appropriate records and can do good single tooth dentistry then you have the skills and knowledge that you need to increase OVD.

This is because a Michigan Splint is actually a removable full mouth reconstruction appliance with ideal occlusion. So if you can do that to a patient, you can use those principles into your restorations.

FIGURE 35a

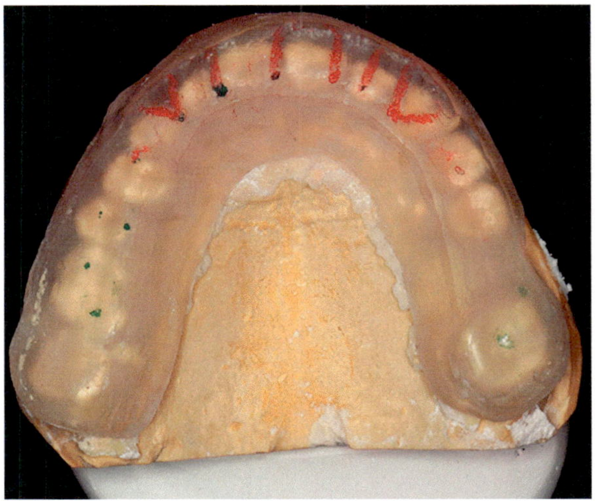

FIGURE 35b

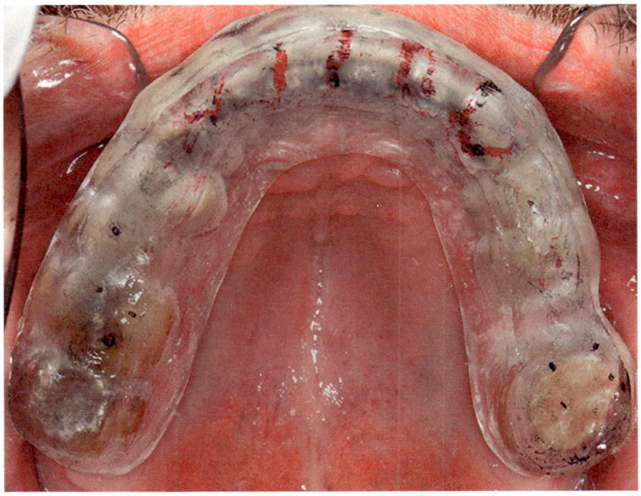

Benefits of increasing OVD

The benefits are three-fold. They are **aesthetic, biomechanical** and **occlusal**.

❖ **Aesthetic benefits**

- You can increase a patient's incisal length freely and give them a nice smile design.
- You can flatten a patient's occlusal plane, which is more visually pleasing.

❖ **Biomechanical benefits:**

- You have control over occlusal forces, which allows you to lengthen the patient's incisor, in turn helping with aesthetics.
- It protects the weakened anterior teeth. For example, when the patient has a deep bite then it can be changed by raising OVD by doing restoration or by orthodontic treatment.
- It helps in creating room for restorative material when you sometimes might not have enough room.

❖ **Occlusal benefits**

- Making the occlusal plane levelled creates less interference.
- Forces are well distributed.
- You get more control during your treatment and more freedom to treat a wide range of cases.

Figure 36a and ***36b*** shows severe tooth wear and deep bite.

FIGURE 36a

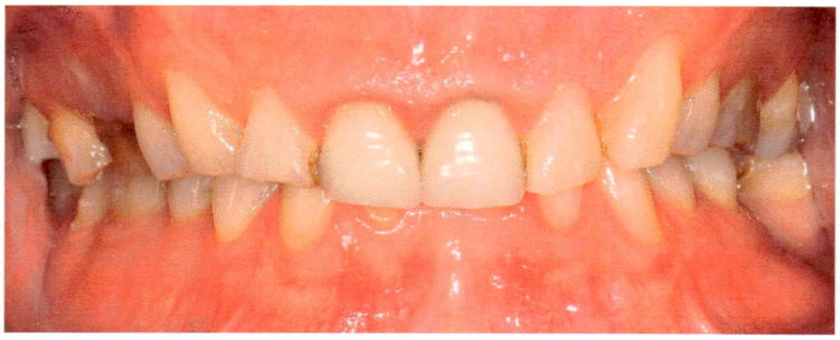

FIGURE 36b

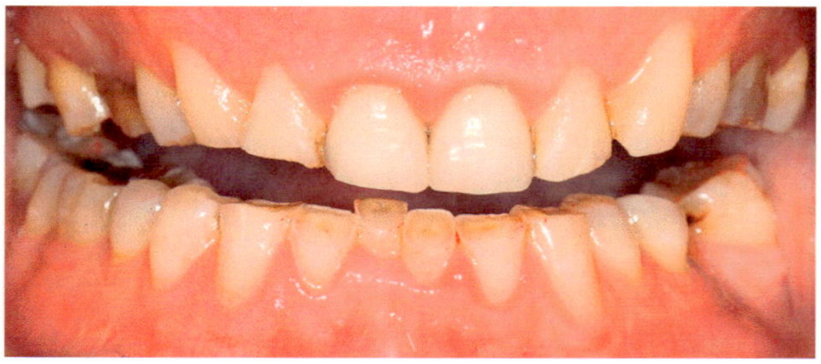

Figure 37 shows broken down posterior restorations.

FIGURE 37

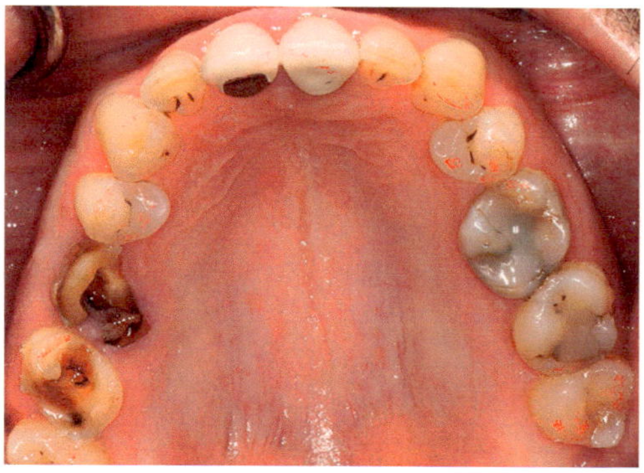

Figures 38a, 38b, 38c and ***38d*** show restoring anterior teeth first and then restoring posterior teeth.

We are going to discuss this step-by-step approach in another chapter. Yet this is just to show you that increasing OVD has given me a lot of space to place an indirect restoration without damaging a patient's teeth. ***Figure 39*** and ***Figure 40*** show the finished result.

FIGURE 38a

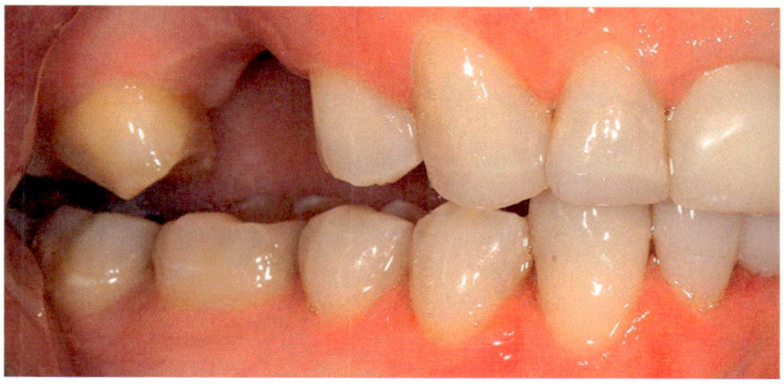

FIGURE 38b

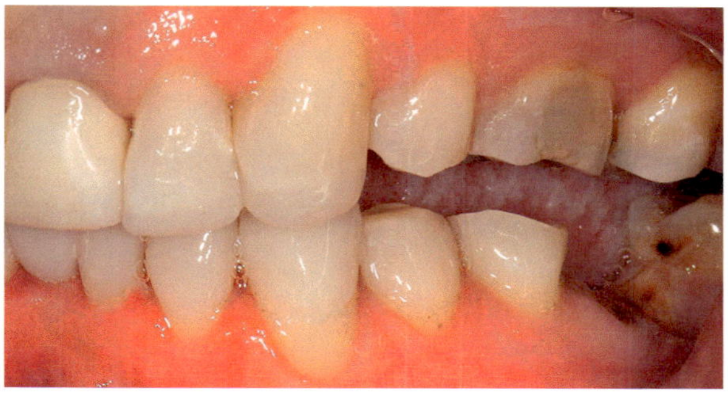

FIGURE 38c

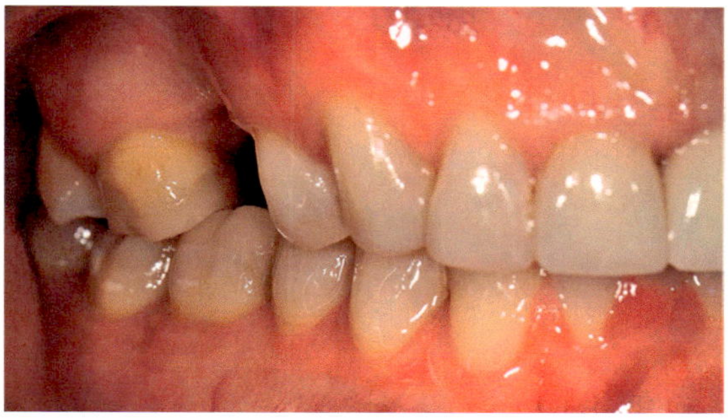

FIGURE 38d

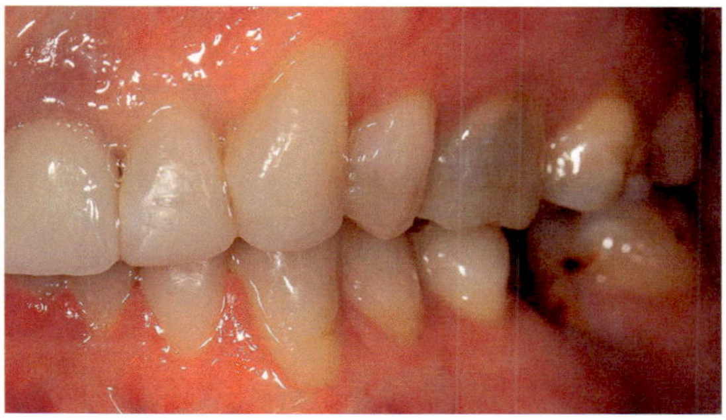

FIGURE 39

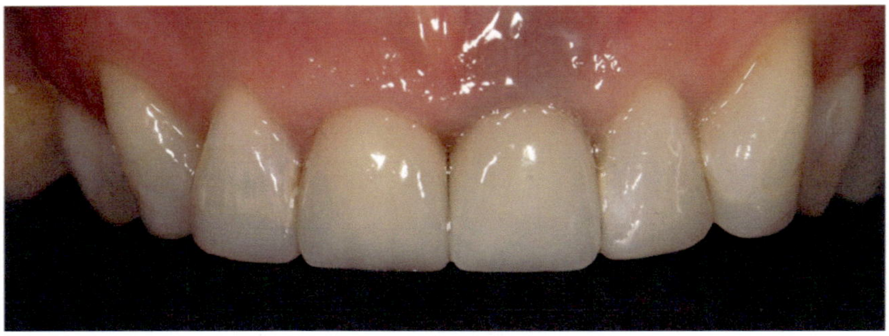

FIGURE 40

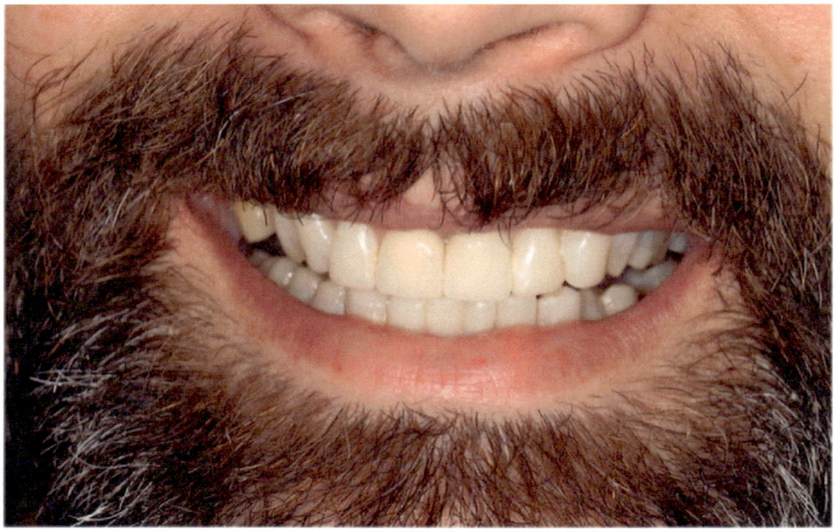

Figure 41 shows another case, one with mild to moderate tooth surface loss.

FIGURE 41

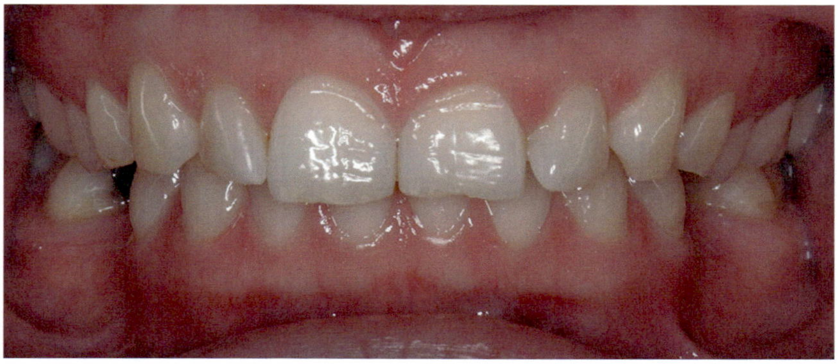

Again, increasing OVD allowed me to do direct restorations to a patient without drilling their teeth. This patient is still young and in her lifetime she will need some of the treatment repeated. Because of that, I need to make sure that I provide her with minimally-invasive treatment. ***Figure 42a*** and ***Figure 42b*** showing before and after results.

FIGURE 42a

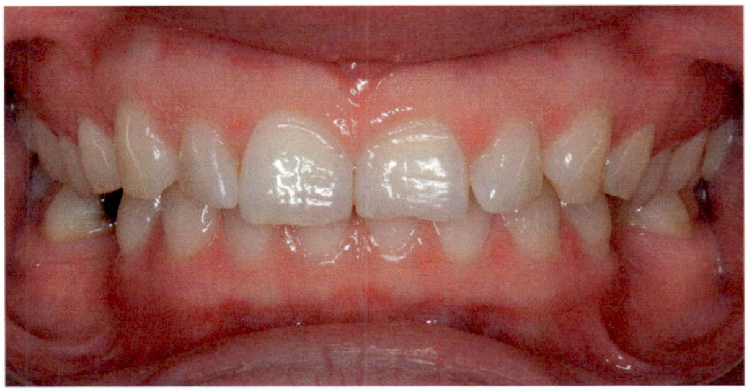

FIGURE 42b

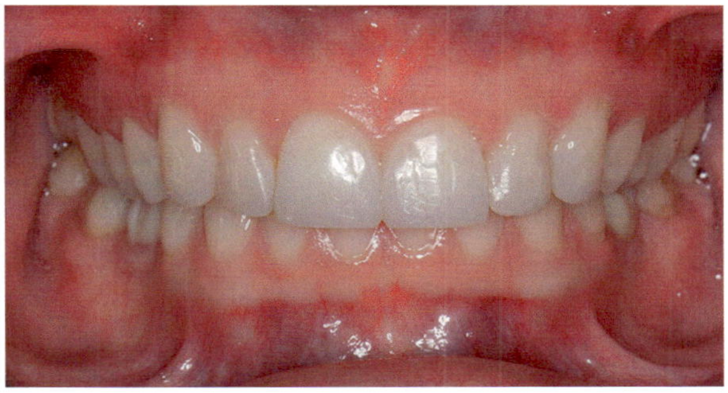

Amount of increase in OVD

- Increasing OVD is very much dependent on the aesthetic and occlusal needs of that patient.
- Anterior teeth usually determine the height of the increase of OVD. This is because if you want to increase OVD posteriorly, let's say by 4mm, it will magnify anteriorly. That's why anterior teeth usually dictate how much of an opening you can make without creating an anterior open bite or very long anterior teeth.
- You can use visual inspection or you can use an articulator in order to assess how much opening you will need. But generally, when I'm doing a clinical assessment, I will ask the patient to open their mouth gradually and stop at a desired OVD, and I'll visualise how my restorations will look, using a patient's mouth as a natural articulator. This helps me in visualising the plan before mounting models.
- Once I've decided what a patient needs, then I will mount a model in an articulator and verify it.

Methods for testing a proposed increase in OVD

Testing the increasing OVD is very important. There are a few ways you can test.

- **Michigan splint (especially if there are TMJ issues)**

  You can use a Michigan Splint, or give a patient a Michigan Splint with the OVD want to raise and let the patient use it for a while, and if the patient is comfortable with it then you can use that as a guide for how much OVD is appropriate and comfortable for that patient.

- **Direct intraoral mock up without preparation of teeth**
  You can use a direct intraoral mockup, where we take the indices of the waxed-up models, and we can then place that into a patient's mouth by using bisacryl material. Then you can let the patient go and test it for a week or so. If the patient is having problems, then you can take all the temporary restorations out, as this process won't have damaged their teeth.

- **Provisional restorations**
  You can use provisional restorations to check OVD. If you have given a patient provisional crowns then you have gone that one step further along. If a patient cannot get used to the crowns then as you have already prepped the teeth for the crowns, you must give them something. That's why you will then have to keep changing the shapes of the teeth until you find the right shape for that patient. You can't go back to a point where the patient has had no treatment done.

  So in my view, a direct intraoral mockup is the best and easiest way to check whether the patient can tolerate their OVD or not, especially when they don't have any TMJ problems.

Choosing guidance

- Make sure that the guidance is shallow and that it reduces the force applied to the teeth and restorations.
- We know from studies that every 10 degree change in the angle of a disclusion means there is a 35 percent change in the force applied. So, if you have a guidance which is, let's say, 10 degrees, and if you change it to 20 degrees to make it steeper, the forces applied on the teeth will be 35 percent more. It's much more magnified, which is why we want shallow guidance to avoid putting too much force on our incisors or canine.

Frequently asked questions

Let's look at some of the questions I am frequently asked.

Why do you need to change the OVD?

OVD can be increased to create space for restorative material, to lengthen a patient's teeth. So if patients come in with shortened teeth but closed spaces, one of the best ways to restore them is by raising OVD.

The other main way to restore them is by doing crown-lengthening and restoring them into existing OVD, but that can be quite invasive.

How much OVD can you increase?

The answer is, as much as a patient can tolerate.

Most of the worries dentists have been related to cases which are edentulous, which work differently. We have a set limit on how much we can raise in an edentulous patient. We need to leave this freeway space of 2 mm, making sure we don't encroach on it.

However, when patients have teeth, it's completely different.

Studies have shown that you can increase to 6-8 mm without having any issues with a patient. Because the patient has proprioception, the teeth have the PDL ligaments which have nerves that connect with the brain, giving you that feedback that you know just indicates a change in dimension.

A patient is much more likely to get used to changes in OVD when they have teeth versus if they have changes in OVD while wearing dentures. So the patient can usually get used to it. However, if the patient has some TMD issues then you need to test that before you give them any definitive restorations.

Do I mount my models in CR or ICP?

Do you really need to mount models in CR? The short answer is yes. When you mount a model in CR, it provides a predictable reference point which you can go back to again and again.

If you mount a model in ICP, you need to prepare for a lot of adjustment because the patient's jaw can relax and the position can change. You can get away with it most of the time without taking this into consideration, but there will almost certainly be times when you will get stuck.

My job is to give you a system which works most of the time. With a little bit more hassle, you get much more predictable results if you mount a model in CR.

How stable are changes in vertical dimensions over time?

There are studies that show the vertical dimension which you increased to goes back to normal because muscles cannot divide and cannot lengthen. Because of that, there will be supraeruption or intrusion, and then the vertical dimension will be the same and the face changes don't happen.

However, there are other studies which show that muscles adapt and lengthen, and then the OVD stays the same.

In any case, even if there is a relapse, patients are unaware of that relapse as it doesn't have any functional issues. And because of that, whether OVD relapses or not doesn't have any implication for you as a restorative dentist.

The only time it does make a difference is when you're doing implant restorations. Let's say you increased the OVD, restored the teeth, and now you're doing an implant restoration. We know that if the OVD settles, all the forces will be loaded onto your implant restorations. That's why it's ideal to do a full mouth reconstruction first.

Change the OVD and restore the implants six months after you've changed it because we know that the majority of the changes happen within those six months. So delay your restoration of the implant until after you've done a full mouth reconstruction.

Will the patient be able to tolerate it?

The answer is test, test, test. Make sure you test this in your Michigan splint, in your diagnostic mock up and in your provisionals. Until you test it, you will never know.

Any TMJ issues or muscle pain?

If you've done a load test as we discussed before and the patient has got no issues, then it's unlikely that the patient is going to have issues after you raised the OVD.

But if there is an issue with load testing then it's highly likely that the patient may not be able to tolerate it. That's why we won't go ahead until the patient's load testing is verified and they are not in pain.

As we discussed, you can use a lucia jig or leaf gauge to do the load test.

What about speech?

Speech - 'S' sounds?

If the patient has an 's' sound then they are lisping, which means they are not enunciating words properly, which could be because of the bulk of the palatal surface.

To adjust this, get the patient's ICP contacts with black or blue articulating paper, then put a red articulating paper and ask the patient to make that sound. Wherever teeth are touching but not at an ICP contact point, you need to adjust it. This should reduce the lisping.

Sometimes, the lower incisors are too long, which means you then need to reduce the length of the lower incisor. That will reduce your OVD.

Speech - 'F' sounds?

This sound is usually not related to a change of OVD. Instead it's usually related to the length of the upper incisor teeth. Therefore, just reduce the length of the upper incisor teeth, and that will help.

How can you check if the teeth have supraerupted?

A way to check this is when a patient is smiling and showing a lot of teeth surface, as that means they have got dento alveolar compensation, which means they have supraerupted. Whereas if patients are not showing that many teeth, that means they have lost OVD, and by increasing OVD it will help you in giving them their smile back.

Limitations

- OVD only changes the dental tissue. It doesn't change the face shape. So if a patient has a collapsed face, it may not make that much difference, unless it's a dramatic change in OVD. You need to communicate that with your patient. Although it is very drastic in denture patients, it is not the case for every dentate patient.
- Increasing OVD is not ideal when a patient has had a dento alveolar compensation, and for those patients orthodontic treatment is the best way forward or sometimes crown-lengthening or orthognathic surgery in extreme cases.
- But usually we start with orthodontic treatment in moving the teeth into that position, because if you just add on to the teeth which are already supraerupted because of dental alveolar compensation, then the occlusal plane will not be flat.

Techniques for changing OVD

- You can make use of a change of freeway space, which means you can encroach into it if it's more than 2mm. As discussed, this is more relevant for dentures.
- You can use trial appliances.
- You can use the TENS appliance.

- You can measure the distance between the cementoenamel junction, and with a free hand build up just open up the patient's bite.
- You can check the patient's facial proportion. Yet as we discussed, it's not always reliable.

All these methods are derived from removable prosthodontics.

My way

So I use two methods when it comes to raising the OVD from a patient's current ICP.

Option 1: I would either raise the OVD in the patient's CO (first point of contact) if I know that the patient may not be able to tolerate too much change. If you restore the patient while they are in CO, the patient's muscle won't have to change or won't have to tolerate much because they already go back into their CO every time they swallow. You can therefore feel sure that the patient will be able to adapt to their new changed OVD.

Option 2: I will raise the OVD in the patient's CR. I will be mounting a model in CR and testing the increase in the patient's mouth via a diagnostic mock up.

Materials used when changing OVD

Let's look at some of the materials you can use when you're changing OVD. What determines which material you're going to use?

The answer is:

- The position of the teeth in the arch.
- The quality of the remaining tooth tissue.
- The patient's wishes. This is because many times patients may want porcelain teeth because they look nice, often not wanting buccal composite veneers. In that case, you may want to adapt your treatment plan to porcelain veneers or crowns depending on what treatment modality is suitable, and where it is.

Available materials

Conventionally we've tended to restore teeth using cast gold onlays and porcelain fused to metal (PFM) for crowns.

However, nowadays, you can use direct composite resin as well as indirect composite resin, combined with adhesive onlays or ceramic onlays.

Direct composite

Direct composites are one of the materials of choice for full mouth reconstruction.

It gives you predictable and beautiful results. ***Figures 43a*** and ***Figure 43b*** show before and after photos of posterior teeth restored using direct composite. ***Figures 44a*** and ***Figure 44b*** show before and after photos of anterior teeth restored using direct composite.

FIGURE 43a

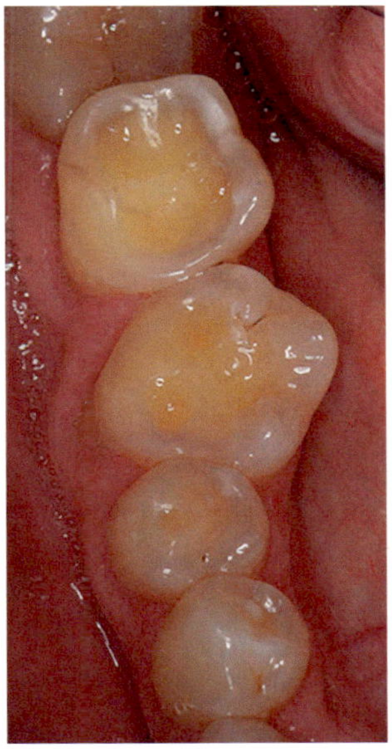

FIGURE 43b

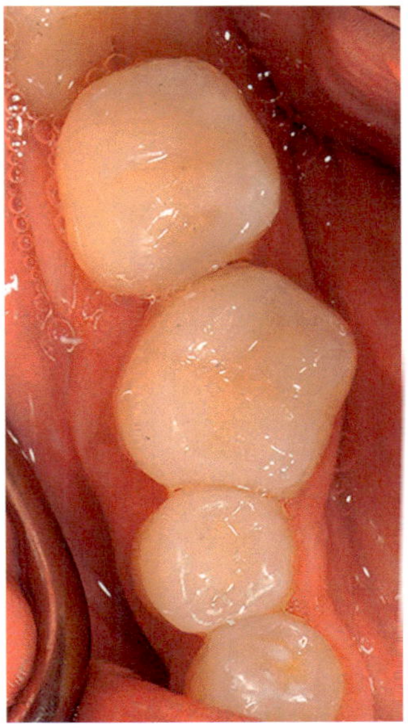

FIGURE 44a

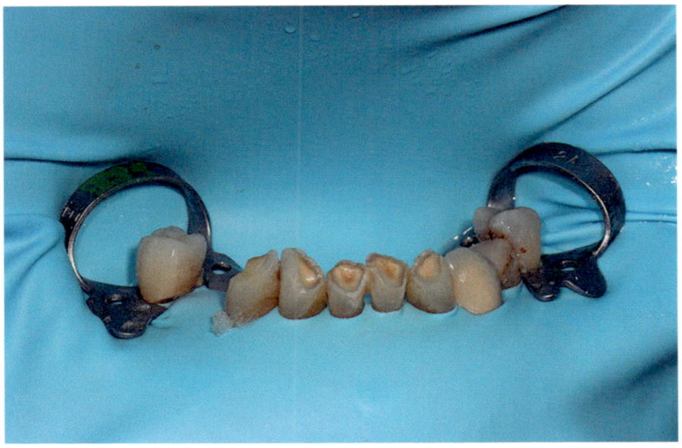

FIGURE 44b

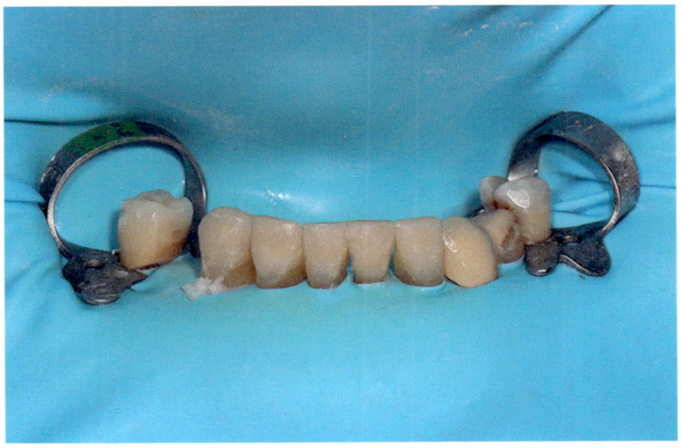

FIGURE 44c

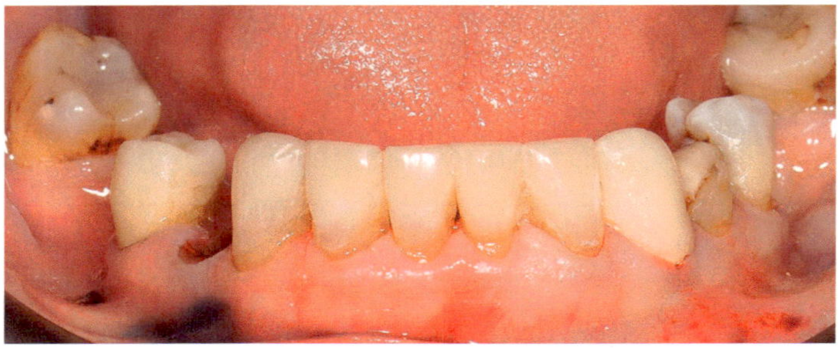

Direct composite - advantages

- It gives you acceptable aesthetic outcomes.
- You can have a non-invasive procedure.
- It may be used as a diagnostic tool to start the treatment first and then convert into an indirect restoration later on.
- It's well-tolerated by pulp and tissues.
- It's minimally invasive to teeth, which is very important.
- It's easy to repair and adjust, which makes it much easier to manage in future.
- It's a cost-effective material.
- A restoration may be applied within a single visit.

Direct composite - disadvantages

- You have accelerated wear due to the nature of the material itself.
- You can get bulk fracture (although this is unlikely to happen if you manage the occlusion well).
- Composite restorations get discoloration. Staining is one of the key drawbacks because it depends on your bonding technique as well as your patient's habits - and the latter is something you don't have any control over.
- It requires moisture control.
- You need a good quality and quantity of enamel.
- It can be complex to do extensive restorations.
- Polymerisation shrinkage.

Indirect composite restorations

Because of that, you can use indirect composite restoration, which avoids some of the disadvantages of direct composite restoration. ***Figure 45a*** and ***Figure 45b*** show before and after photos of the case restored with composite.

FIGURE 45a

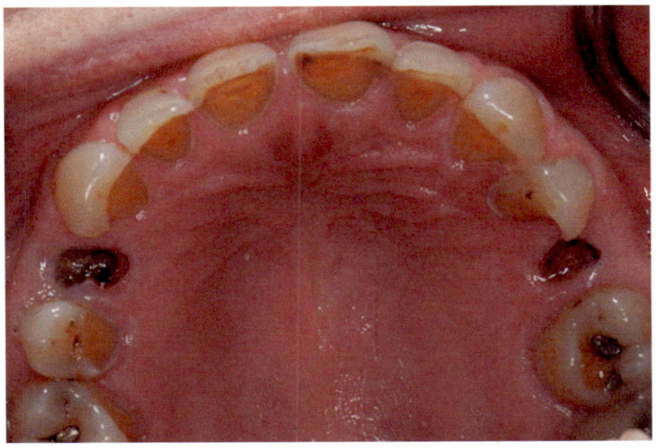

FIGURE 45b

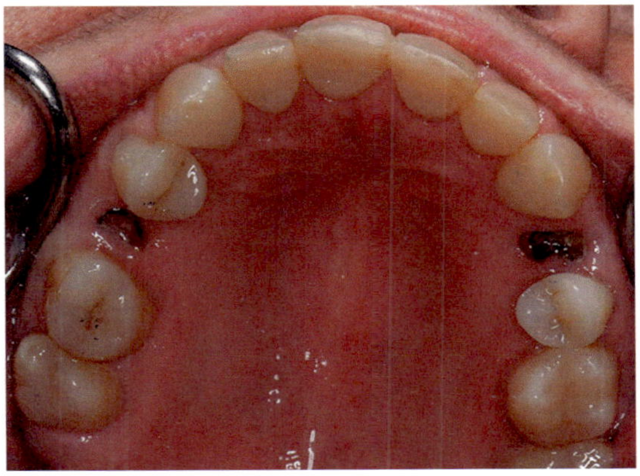

Indirect composite - advantages

- You get a very accurate fit.
- There's minimal wear because of the material's properties.
- It's protective towards any residual surface.
- It's suitable for posterior restoration. When doing this I use a material called BelleGlass from Kerr,or CAD/CAM composite blocks called Cerasmart from Dentaplysirona.
- It's placed supragingivally, which preserves the patient's periodontal health.
- Minimal tooth preparation is required because composite can be done in a thin section, especially when you're bonding it with a heated restorative composite.

Indirect composite - disadvantages

- There is a need for copious amounts of enamel (as with any bonding).
- Sometimes there are difficulties when placing provisional restorations.
- Increased cost.

Adhesive ceramic restorations

The third modality is ceramic restorations. They often look very nice because they are adhesive or cemented crowns. ***Figure 46a*** and ***Figure 46b*** showing before and after photos of the case completed using ceramics.

FIGURE 46a

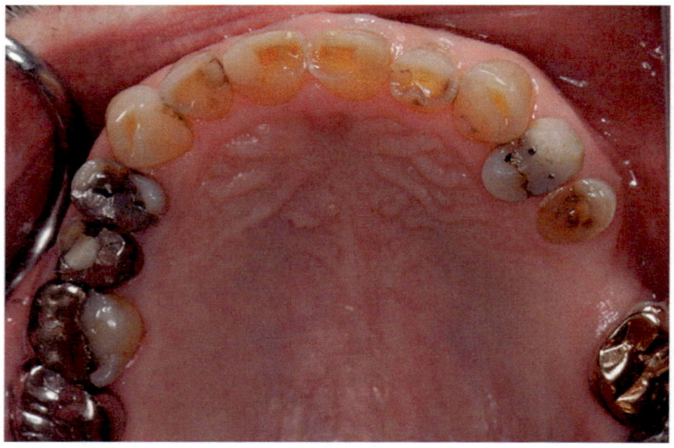

FIGURE 46b

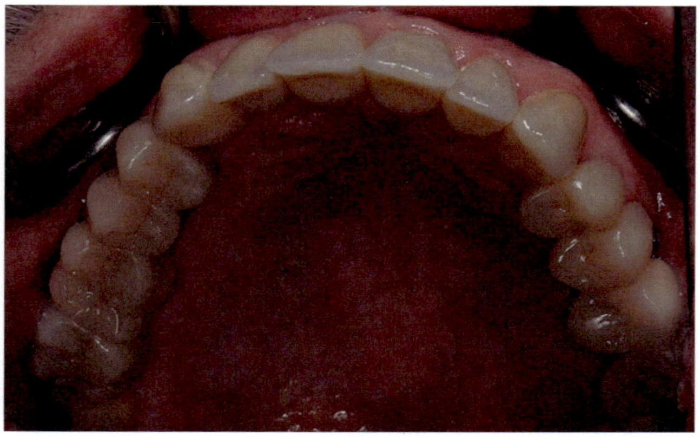

Adhesive ceramic restorations - advantages

- Superior aesthetics.
- Good resistance to abrasion.
- Lower relative surface-free energy compared to resin composites, making it less susceptible to staining and very easy to maintain if they're done really nicely.
- Higher level of gingival tissue tolerance.

In the long term, porcelain and direct veneers or direct restorations may need more maintenance, even though there are many advantages.

Adhesive ceramic restorations - disadvantages

- These restorations can be brittle and prone to fracture, and if they break it's very difficult to repair them. You will probably have to have a new restoration made, and if a patient is bruxist there is likelihood that they will subject them to a lot of force.
- They are also more abrasive towards the opposing teeth. If you're working on the anterior teeth - let's say canine to canine upper crowns - and you're doing lower composite buildups, your composite buildups are going to wear down much quicker. It's why I prefer a sandwich technique where I do composite buildups on the lower teeth, a palatal

composite build up, and then buccal veneers on the upper arch. This means you can get the best of both worlds.

- As we discussed, these restorations are difficult to repair intraorally, and difficult to adjust.
- They are susceptible to degradation and wear from acidic environments.
- They are costly.

Having analysed the disadvantages, you need to really weigh them up against the advantages of composite and porcelain.

Usually if a patient is much older I prefer porcelain because it will involve less maintenance. If patients are very young and a porcelain restoration will damage their teeth, then I will use a composite restoration. Patients always need to be told that composite is an interim restoration only. At some point in their lifetime they will have to have more work done, most likely followed up by an indirect restoration.

2.3 DAHL Principle

We know that from a survey conducted among adults in the UK in 1998 that two thirds have some sort of anterior wear, while ten percent have moderate or severe tooth wear. And this is getting worse and hence 20 years later we can only imagine the numbers rising.

Cases such as that in ***Figure 47a*** and ***Figure 47b*** have become quite routine in general dental practice. Some sort of tooth wear can be found in patients as young as 14 or 18, or as late as 70 or 80 years old. ***Figure 47a*** is a 70 years old gentleman and ***Figure 47b*** is a 23 years old girl.

FIGURE 47a

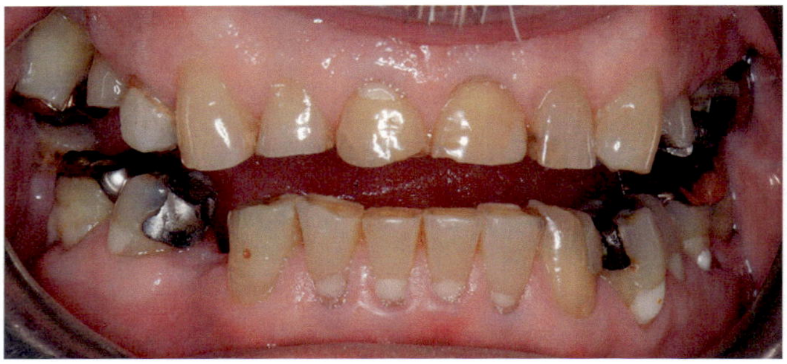

FIGURE 47b

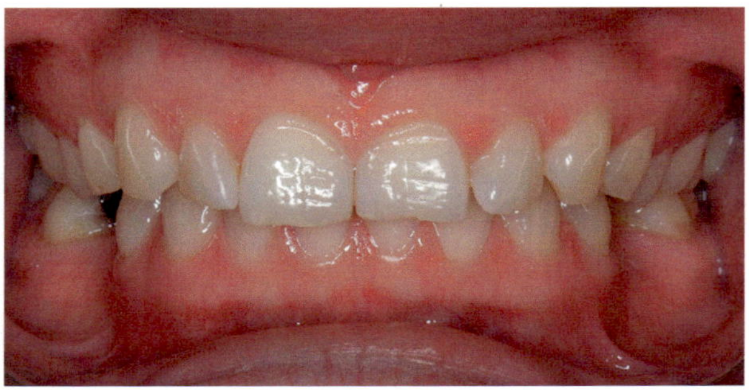

When to treat?

This is a controversial topic because some people would argue that as soon as the dentine starts getting exposed, you need to treat those teeth. Otherwise the dentin will wear down more rapidly than the enamel, as studies have shown many times.

Yet you will find localised wear that some of the dentists are not willing to treat because it can be invasive or extensive. Supraeruption or dento-alveolar compensation can then happen in these cases if dentine has been left alone and ultimately the space closes. And once that space is closed, the clinician will struggle to restore those teeth as you do not have restorative space. The occlusal contacts will still be maintained because of the dentoalveolar compensation.

Treatment options

What are our treatment options in such cases, where you have localised anterior tooth wear but the contacts are completely maintained and there is no space for you to place any restoration?

Option 1: You can try and conform to ICP, **creating a space by grinding the teeth and restoring them with crowns**. However, that is much more destructive than doing nothing, so I generally wouldn't recommend it.

Option 2: You could do **crown-lengthening and place a crown** on the tooth. But again, this is much more destructive than normal treatment modalities.

Option 3: You could do **a reorganised approach by increasing the OVD** and doing a full mouth reconstruction. But again, if the posterior teeth are intact then that leads to unnecessary treatment on those posterior teeth.

Option 4: You can give patients an **orthodontic appliance** and try and move the teeth, which is a much more valid way.

Option 5: You can give the patient a **DAHL appliance** which is essentially an orthodontic appliance that could be removable or fixed or you can do a direct build up using the same concept.

Nowadays it is more likely if you are using a **DAHL** concept that you'll do a direct composite build-up using **DAHL** principles.

What is the DAHL concept?

The DAHL concept refers to relative axial tooth movement that is observed when a localised appliance or localised restoration is placed in a supraocclusion. You are placing the restoration high and in contact. The occlusion will eventually re-establish full arch contact.

Relevant studies suggest a 94 to 100 percent success rate in doing this type of treatment modalities.

There are other phrases that have been used to describe the DAHL principle, such as 'minor axial tooth movement', 'fixed orthodontic intrusion appliances', 'localised interocclusal space creation', or 'relative axial tooth movement'. But they all describe the same thing.

A removable appliance

The DAHL principle was popularised in 1975. It was described by other dentists before but DAHL is the one who really popularised the principle of space creation by giving the patient a removable appliance.

The patient used to wear the removable appliance in a state of high contact. Only the teeth which DAHL wanted to move were in contact, mainly the upper canine to canine. By doing that, he saw a supraeruption of the posterior teeth of around 60% and an intrusion of the anterior teeth of around 40 percent.

After he created the space, he then placed indirect restoration like crowns or gold palatal backings on the palatal aspects because at that time composites weren't very good.

This removable appliance was then improvised by fixing a Maryland bridge with just wings on canine to canine. However, the problem was that when the removal of these wings became very difficult, dentists started causing iatrogenic problems by damaging teeth. Hence, now we are mainly considering composite build ups in a supra eruption. Use of composite has made this technique much more convenient and easy to use.

This treatment is more effective in younger patients because the tooth movement is better. However, it can be used regardless of a patient's age.

You do see some condylar repositioning happening during the treatment, and the best way to know whether that's happened or not is when you see posterior contacts within a couple of weeks. That means you're definitely seeing condylar repositioning because teeth don't move that quickly.

DAHL principle - indications

One of the main indicators for the use of the DAHL principle is when you see localised anterior wear where the posterior teeth are intact, with most of these cases being erosive cases. Because they're erosive cases, you tend to see much more rapid wear. The patient will have lost OVD as a result, and this is the ideal time to apply the DAHL principle and use the **DAHL** technique.

DAHL principle - contraindications

Unfortunately, there are more contraindications than indications.

- If a patient's teeth are periodontally involved with bone loss, then you cannot use the DAHL technique.
- It is not recommended if a patient has worn posterior teeth. If a patient has severe attrition of the anterior and posterior teeth, then they need a full mouth reconstruction.
- If a patient has severe crowding or inter-arch discrepancies and as a result of this, teeth do not move that easily and hence DAHL treatment may not work. Similarly, if a patient's teeth are quite flared out and you cannot get that 90-degree axial loading, you cannot treat those patients using the DAHL technique as you may move teeth in unwanted directions.
- Obviously, if a patient has an anterior open bite then you cannot do it.
- If a patient has any TMD problems, then you need to make sure, as with any full mouth reconstruction, that the patient is cured or the symptoms have gone.
- Also, if a patient has a class 3 occlusion then doing the DAHL technique is going to be nearly impossible.

What are the materials you can use when applying this principle?

You can use:

- direct composite
- indirect composite
- all-ceramic crowns
- ceramic or gold palatal veneers

These are all the modalities.

Whenever dentists use these materials or apply the DAHL principle, two questions frequently come up: how much space can I create, and how long is it going to take before teeth come into contact?

Space creation

With regards to the space creation, we know from studies you could create up to a 1.4 to 4.7 mm space but if you keep it to 1 to 4 mm then it's safer. You can measure this very easily with a caliper ruler measuring distance between gingival margins of upper and lower central incisors before and after wax up. This is also one of the easiest ways to measure the increase of OVD once you have done actual build up too.

Time

Time-wise it can take anything between three to six months. However, I tell patients that it can take up to 18 months according to some studies.

Usually however, most of the tooth movement happens in three to six months. I do warn patients that if their teeth haven't come into contact, then they will need some restoration for the posterior teeth. So the patient needs to be aware of that and the associated fees.

Criteria when applying the DAHL principle

- If the upper cingulum is intact and it's just the lower anteriors that are worn, and if I can get a lower anterior buildup and a 90-degree axial loading of the upper anterior, then I can just build the lower anterior teeth.

  However, if the upper anteriors are also worn then it's better to build the upper and lower anterior teeth.

- We need to make sure that the loading is in the axial direction otherwise you may notice flaring of the teeth. If the loading is not in the **axial** direction (as shown in ***Figure 67***) then you start seeing more chipping or breakage of the restoration.
- Keep the total build-up as we discussed up to 4 mmm. You could add 2 mm on the upper and 2 mm the lower.
- How much are you going to add between that 1 to 4 mm mark? It will depend on how much overbite you're going to get. If you are maintaining around an overlap of the teeth of around 20 to 30 percent, then that's ideal and as it's what you're going to aim for when you're building the teeth up.
- **Always include the front six teeth as a minimum.** If you include eight teeth (so four teeth on either side), then aesthetically it looks much better. However, at minimum you will need to include six teeth because those canines are really important when guiding the teeth and taking on the forces.

Figure 48 illustrates well what I mean by axial loading or axial force.

You don't want forces to go where the red lines are. Instead you want them in that green arrow zone. This is really important to communicate to your technician.

FIGURE 48

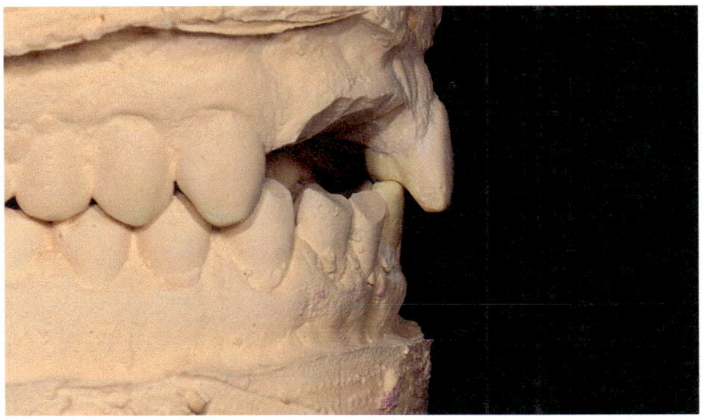

Figure 49a, Figure, 49b and ***Figure 50*** show the correct shape of the palatal build ups - the upper right central incisor is the correct way to build these teeth up (see green arrow). It's not natural-looking and hence technicians have a tendency to build teeth like the left central incisor, without the platform. But this will not work if you're doing DAHL technique. You need to communicate that to the technician.

FIGURE 49a

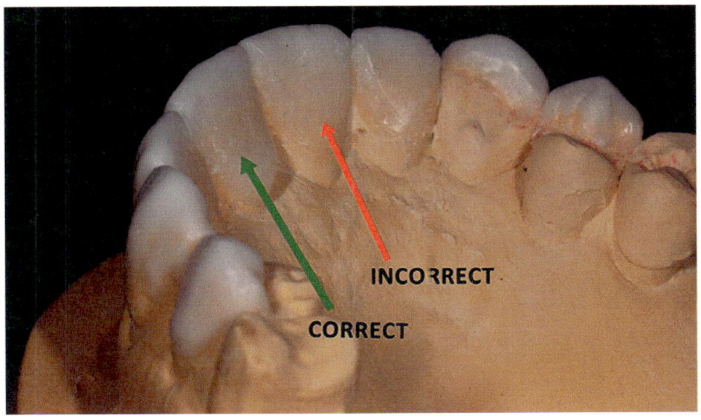

FIGURE 49b

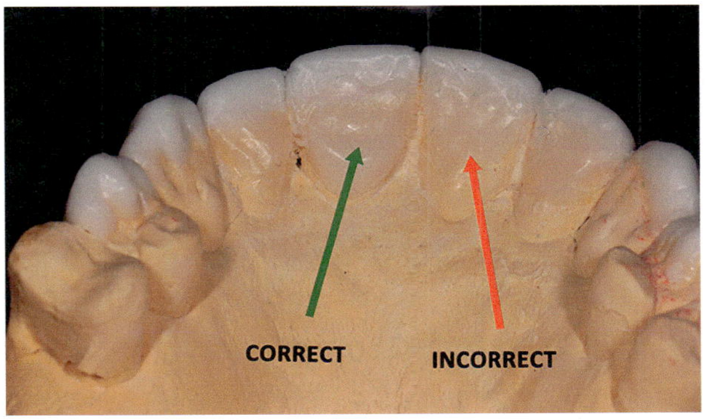

FIGURE 50

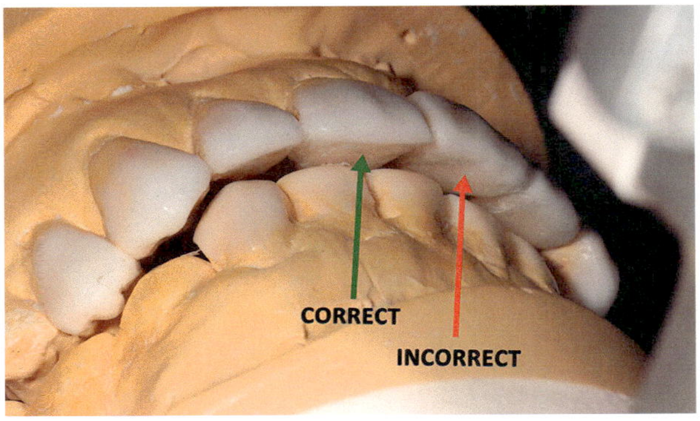

DAHL design

You are aiming to have mutually-protected anterior occlusion:

Which means:

- canine guidance with heavy ICP contacts on canines,
- lighter contacts on incisors,
- axial loading of the forces,
- shallow guidance when patients move their jaw forwards and laterally,
- immediate posterior disclusion, although you will have posterior disclusion because you've raised the OVD (unless there is some supra-eruption).

One stage vs two stage

Another question many dentists ask me is whether they should have a one-stage (straight to final restoration) or two-stage (provisional restoration first and then final restoration once space is closed) approach to DAHL? As we will see, it depends on whether you're doing a direct restoration or an indirect restoration.

Direct restorations

If you're going to do a direct restoration, then it's going to be composite. Just build the teeth up into that definitive shape and form because you can always add just the composite. Of course, you need to carry out a mock-up before you do any build-ups. But you can build DAHL restorations in the final shape and form using composite after mock up and let the teeth supraerupt and intrude. This is a one stage technique.

Indirect restorations

However, if you're doing **indirect restorations** like crowns, then the problem is that once you've done the crowns between canine to canine or premolar to premolar but you don't know how exactly the supraeruption of the posterior and the intrusion of the anterior is going to happen. Often you may have to adjust those restorations.

Yet if you adjust them, you will cause a possible weakening of the restoration, including perforation and micro leakage or chipping of the porcelain, loss of glaze, you may even cause sensitivity of the teeth or lose the restoration.

Therefore, you need to make sure that you have assessed everything. Because of that, I do not go straight to indirect restorations.

If my final plan consists of indirect restorations, then I'll do a two-stage technique where I will build a patient's palatal aspect and incisal edges using composite, and then once everything settles, I will possibly place veneers on the anteriors. If the patient wants a more cosmetic result, or even if you think they need a crown, then that's the point where you would do the crown. At the very least you need to keep the provisional crowns and let the teeth DAHL before you replace them with final crowns.

Monitoring

- Once you have treated the patient, you need to monitor them every two weeks in the beginning and then every month afterwards, until teeth are settled. Every two weeks you need to review the contact points. If a patient has very heavy contact on their incisors, then you need to reduce that load and keep the contact heavy on the canine.
- If there is a posterior interference and you haven't raised the bite enough, with the patient hitting the posterior **teeth while in function**, then you may need to adjust the posterior teeth. This may happen due to the condylar seating because teeth won't supererupt in two weeks. Again, getting consent is very important.
- You can use IPR for the posterior teeth to speed up their movement. If a patient's posterior contacts are quite tight, use a yellow IPR strip to lighten the contacts. Then it's easier for them to supraerupt and not get stuck because of the tight contact.
- Use of the anterior Essix retainer can relieve you of the worry that they will break your restoration.

I never had any issue with my restorations and you won't either if the occlusion is right and they will last without problems. If you're worried, you can give the patient a sectional Essix retainer just to cover your newly restored teeth (canine to canine or premolar to premolar). However, the patient must stop wearing that as soon as the posterior teeth are starting to come into contact. Otherwise, they'll start developing an anterior open bite. You need to make sure that it's very delicately managed and monitored regularly.

Summary

The DAHL principle works very well in young patients with minor to moderate tooth wear with intact posterior teeth. However, case selection is the key whenever you're doing this type of treatment.

2.4 Steps Involved in Simple Adhesive Full Mouth Reconstruction

We're now going to discuss the step-by-step protocol for full mouth direct adhesive reconstruction cases.

Treatment flow for adhesive direct full mouth reconstructions

Step 1: Treatment planning

- Comprehensive assessment.
- Impression and records.
- Mounting models in CR/CO or ICP (which is very rare as usually we mount a model in CR or CO).
- Diagnostic wax up.
- Trying out the mock-up of that diagnostic wax up.

Step 2: Anterior build-ups

- Upper and lower anterior definitive restoration.
- Stabilisation of the posterior teeth.

Step 3: Posterior build-ups and maintenance

- Restoring posterior teeth (one side at a time or one arch at a time).
- Maintaining and protecting your restorations.
- Providing the patient with some maintenance options.

Treatment flow for adhesive direct full mouth reconstructions

Please be aware that in this book we are concentrating on DIRECT build ups and if you are planning to do indirect full mouth reconstructions using crowns, bridges or onlays, then the protocol will be different.

Step-by-step protocol

So, let's look at this case in ***Figure 51a*** and ***Figure 51b.*** A patient came to me with minor to moderate tooth wear, mainly anterior, upper anterior and then posterior.

FIGURE 51a

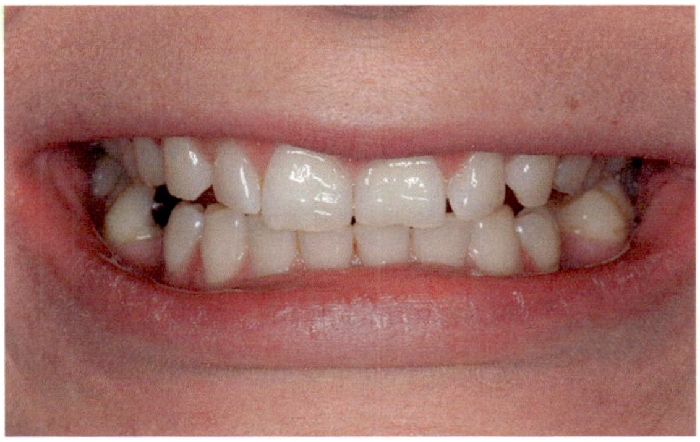

FIGURE 51b

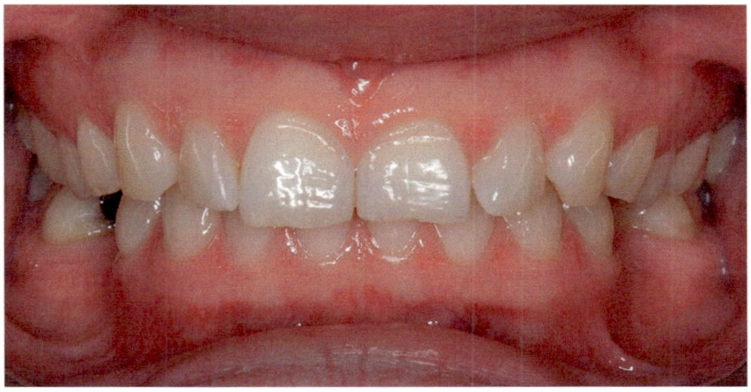

If you look at some of the premolars in ***Figure 52a***, they have quite a lot of wear. Although the photos don't fully show, all the dentine was exposed in the posterior teeth because she used to drink a lot of fizzy drinks and hold it in her mouth, which has caused a lot of wear***. Figure 52b*** showing very mild lower teeth wear.

FIGURE 52a

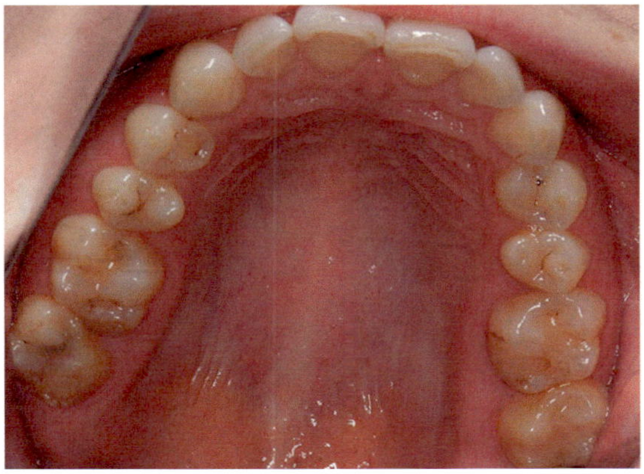

FIGURE 52b

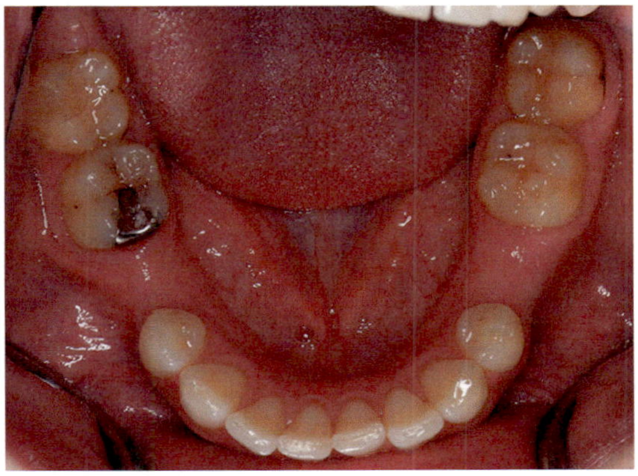

We're now going to examine the step-by-step protocol for planning this case.

Mindset

Before we proceed however, we need to address the mindset you will need going forward.

A dentist's mindset is really important. You need to have the self-belief to know that you can do full mouth reconstructions because sometimes general dental practitioners feel that they cannot do full mouth reconstructions if they are not specialists.

Yet adhesive full mouth reconstruction is very straightforward if you apply the principles I discuss in this book, and if you have done your treatment planning properly. You just need to challenge any self-limiting beliefs.

You need to ask a question: why are you doing full mouth reconstruction? If you're doing it just for the money, then there are better ways to earn money and I would suggest you look for other ways.

But if you really want to give that patient a nice smile and you like a challenge, then full mouth reconstruction is for you.

Also, ask yourself if you are comfortable doing single-tooth dentistry. If you're struggling to do single-tooth dentistry - bonding or onlays or crowns - then you need to really master that first before you end up doing a full mouth reconstruction case. Otherwise, you'll be making the same mistake repeatedly in the same patient when you're doing bonding or indirect restorations.

Therefore, make sure you invest in yourself. This means investing in new instruments or learning new skills and taking the time to implement them.

And last but not the least, get a mentor.

I'm always here if you need someone to talk to but if not me then have someone to talk to who has done more of this work than you so that person can guide you and share their experiences. That advice will help to steer you in the right direction.

If you feel you need support, please feel free to join my Free facebook group called 'Full mouth reconstruction for GDPs' by scanning the code below:

Adhesive full mouth reconstruction - doing direct build-ups step by step procedure

I'm going to describe each appointment for a full mouth reconstruction case in detail. However, you need to take these appointments as steps rather than as a prescriptive road map because the numbering often does not matter, e.g. sometimes it takes two appointments to complete a step. So let's look at all the appointments (steps) you need to carry out full mouth reconstruction. They are listed below.

Appointment 1 – checkup

Currently, I only see patients on a referral basis, but when I began doing full mouth reconstructions, all my patients used to be patients I have seen for checkups. So initially, those checkups used to be 20 minutes and afterwards, if I felt that the patient needed a comprehensive treatment plan then I would reschedule that appointment at a later date for a longer appointment for a further assessment and a discussion. I would tell patients that there are many things going on in their mouth, and if they were interested in doing something about that and keeping their teeth in their mouth for as long as possible then I would need to see them once more to explain exactly what could be done. That way I could help them avoid further degradation of their teeth.

Appointment 2 - treatment planning (Creating a Plan)

The second appointment involves a full mouth assessment. As we discussed in a previous section, listen to the patient's concerns, understand their goals, do a clinical assessment, a radiographic assessment, a tooth by tooth assessment, take a lot of photographs, and if you need to, do intraoral scanning and mount the diagnostic model. Tell the patient about your concerns at the same time.

I don't often tend to do diagnostic wax ups before giving patients some sort of an estimate. It's very important that they understand what your rough estimates are before you ask them to invest any further.

Otherwise, the patient may be taken by surprise if you, after diagnostic wax up, quote them thousands of pounds. This may come as a shock to patients if they do not have any idea of the rough fees. Therefore, you need to give the patient a realistic idea during that appointment.

Once you have this information, you're going to create a treatment plan. You're then going to work on the stabilization phase and make sure all the caries have been removed, periodontal and endodontic treatments have been carried out, if this hasn't been done already.

Appointment 3 - taking records

You will now be seeing the patient for record taking purposes. To do this, you will take impressions, use a facebow, and take CR records to mount a model in CR and ICP. Remember, you mount the model in CR or CO if you need to carry out a wax up and checking of ICP to CO slide and in ICP if you want to do an occlusal assessment.

In ***Figure 53a, Figure 53b*** and ***Figure 53c*** you can see a **facebow** record using putty and bite registration material for partially dentate patients.

FIGURE 53a

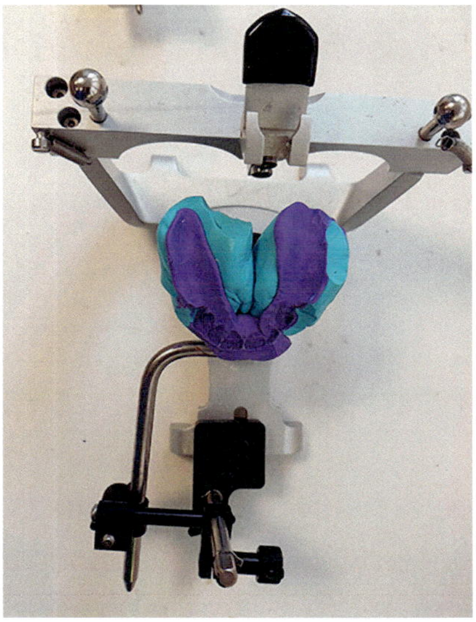

FIGURE 53b

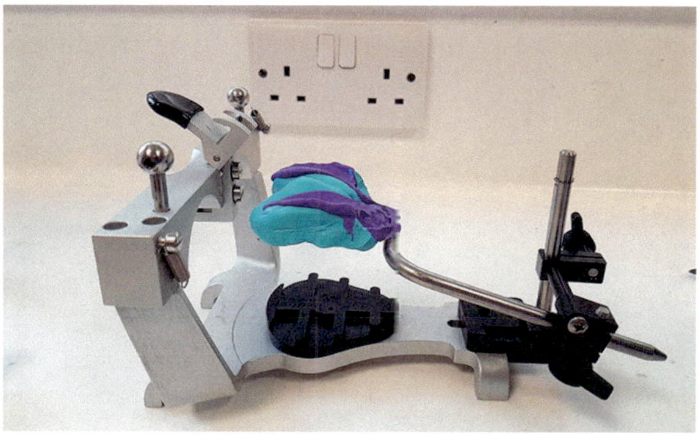

FIGURE 53c

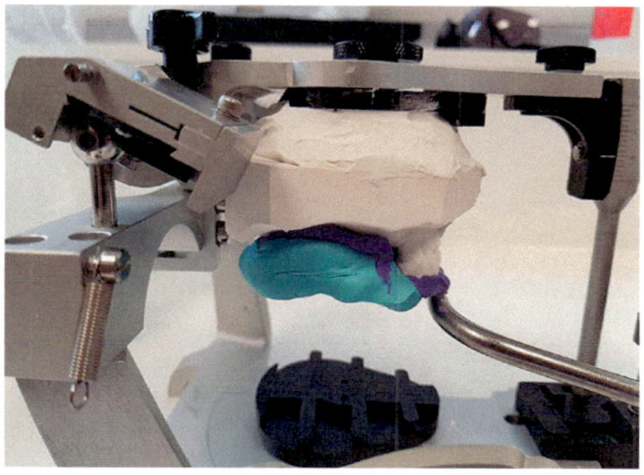

In ***Figure 54*** the **interocclusal records** are taken with a lucia jig, and I've used **a hard bite registration material.**

FIGURE 54

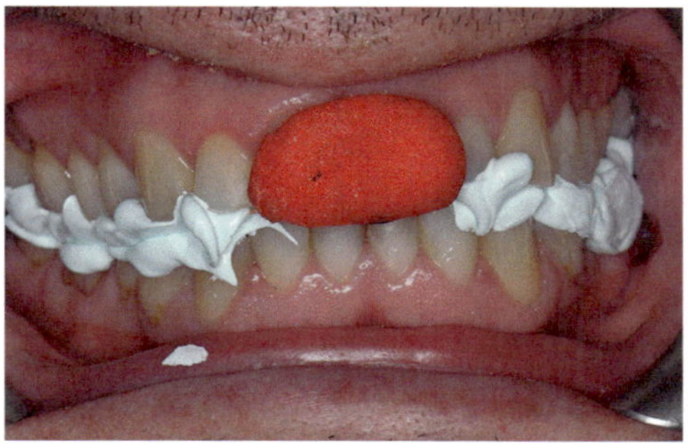

Then we will mount the model and verify our mounting as shown in ***Figure 55a*** use of impression compound and tempbond to verify the accuracy of the model and ***Figure 55b*** showing mounted maxillary models. ***Figure 55c*** shows 3 interocclusal records and ***Figure 55d*** shows mounted maxillary and mandibular models.

FIGURE 55a

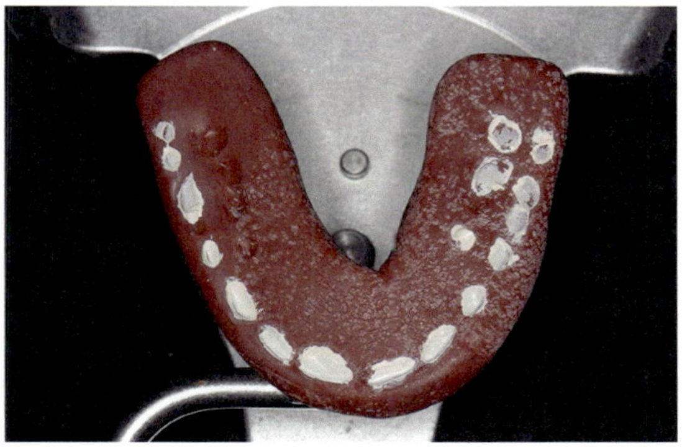

FIGURE 55b

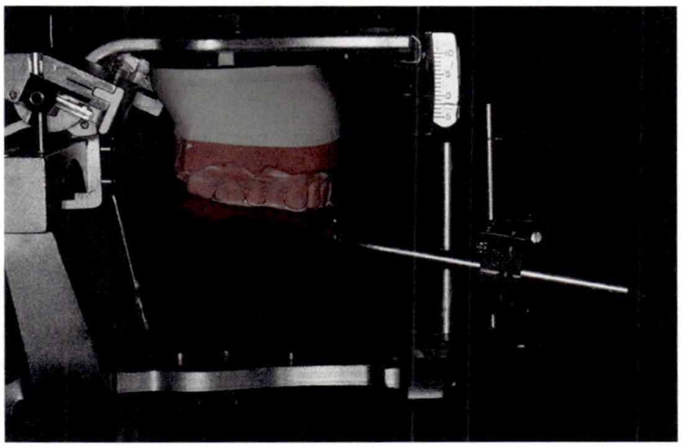

FIGURE 55c

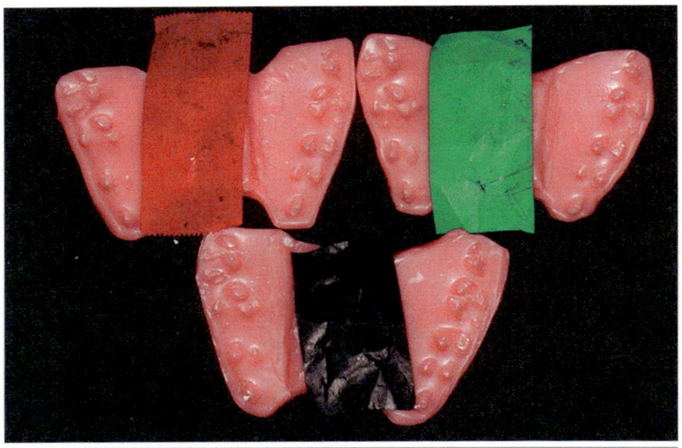

FIGURE 55d

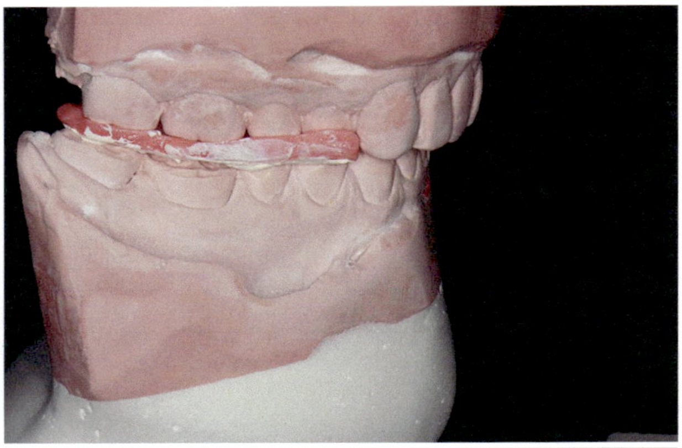

Figures 56a and ***Figure 56b*** show a patient with teeth wear and in need of treatment planning.

FIGURE 56a

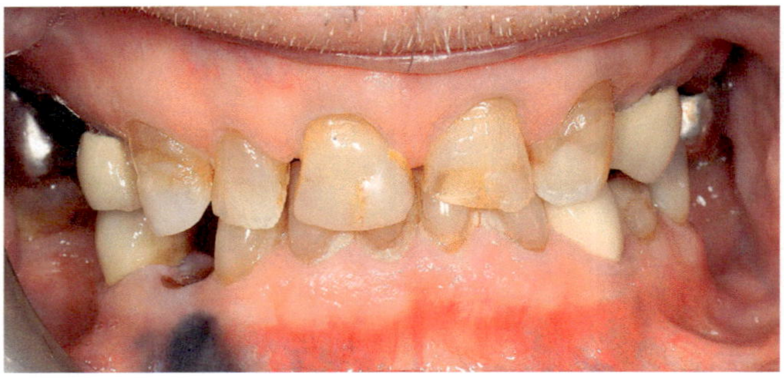

FIGURE 56b

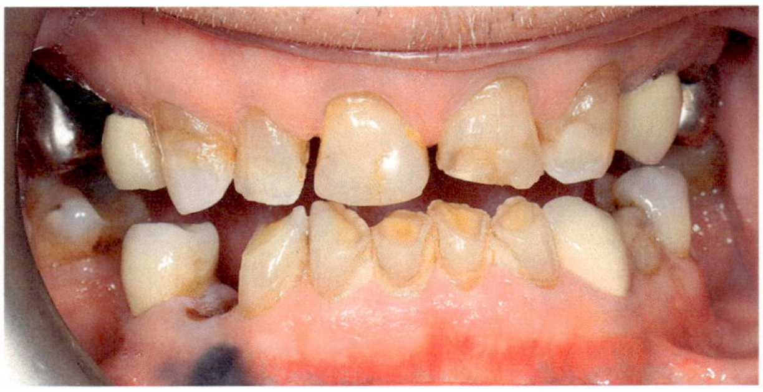

In this case I have used **moyco** beauty wax as a material to take the interocclusal records, and you can see in ***Figures 57a, Figure 57b*** and ***Figure 57c*** how nicely it fits.

FIGURE 57a

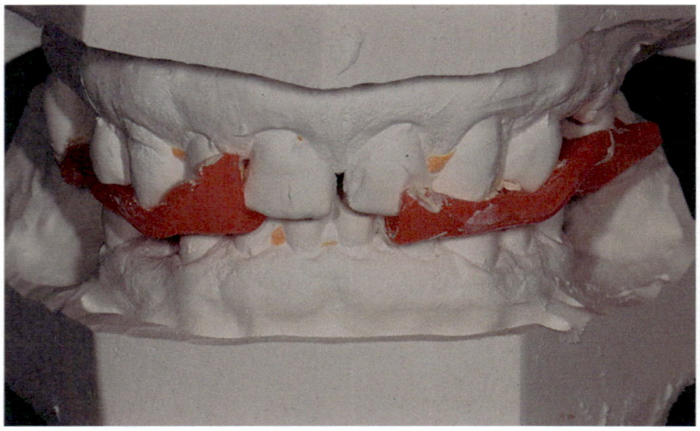

FIGURE 57b

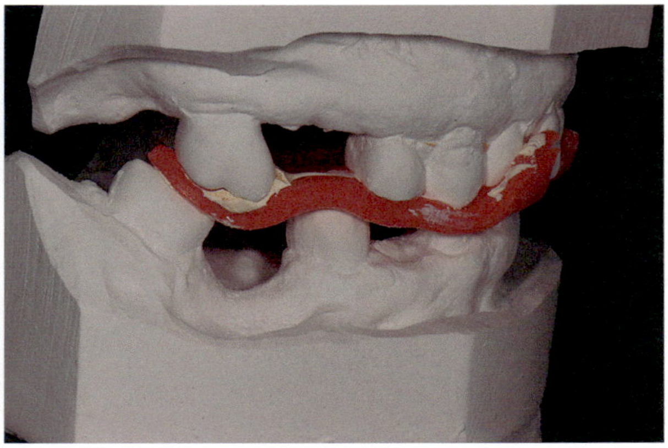

FIGURE 57c

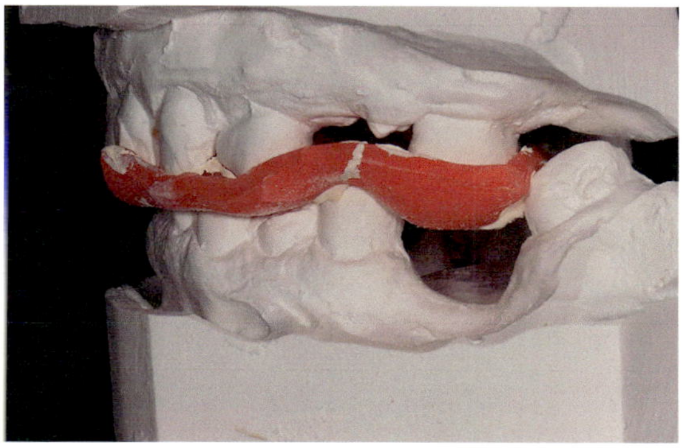

In ***Figure 58a*** you can see the first point of contact. In ***Figure 58b*** what I'm trying to visualise is the occlusal plane by opening the articulator at a desired OVD (on the right hand side picture). You'll need to gauge how much opening will be necessary to make the occlusal plane flat.

FIGURE 58a

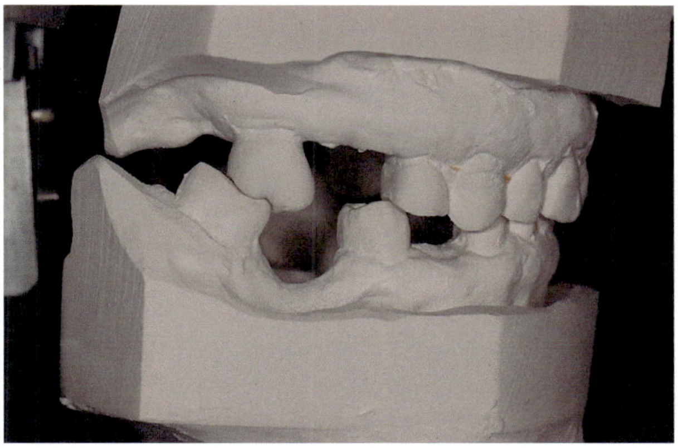

FIGURE 58b

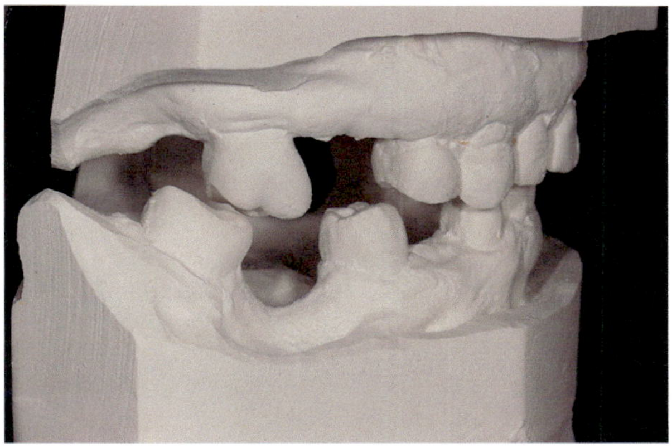

This is relevant to our discussion about limiting factors. The patient's lower right second premolar (in ***Figure 58b***) has a new, good-quality crown that has just been fitted. We are trying to visualise whether it's possible for us to keep that crown.

This is why it's very important to assess the mounted model before the technician has done a diagnostic wax up. You will need to guide the technician as to how much of an opening is needed, how much wax they need to put on the lower arch, and how much wax they need to put on the upper arch. Before you guide technician, however, you need to know what the mounting will look like. So once the models are mounted, you need to make an assessment. Ideally, mark with a pencil the exact surfaces you would like your technician to place wax on and set the pin height to advise the technician about raise in OVD.

Figure 59a showing left side of the view with the position of the teeth after pin was dropped so models are in CO. In ***Figure 59b*** and you can see how much of an opening I have to make to get the plane to be flatter. Even then that tooth (upper left first molar) which is supraerupted is going to cause some issues. It will be impossible to correct the lower left second molar in the plane without orthodontic treatment. So I need to make sure that I convey that to the patient if they have said that they don't want any **enameloplasty** for orthodontic treatment.

FIGURE 59a

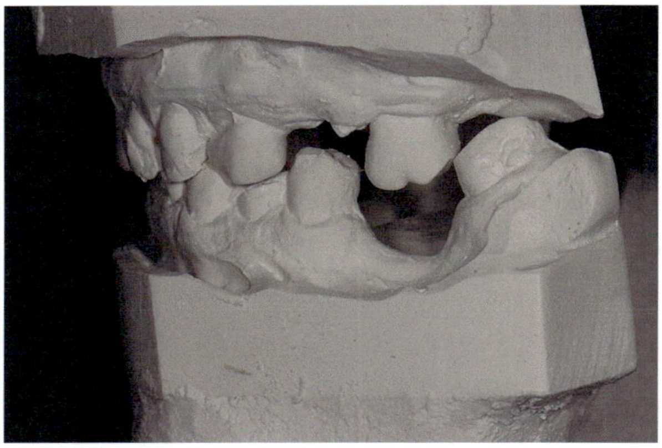

FIGURE 59b

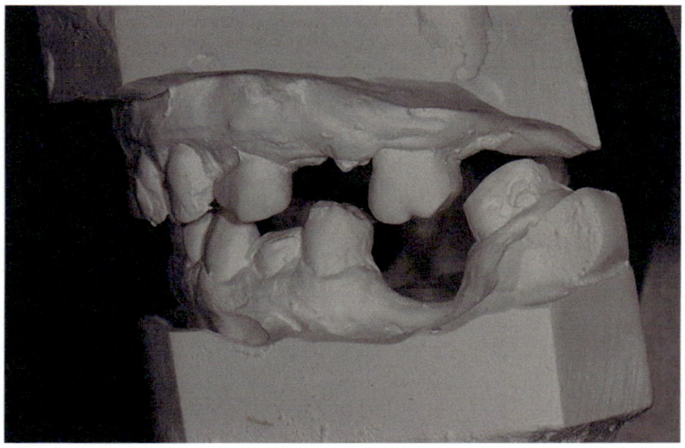

Figures 60, 61a, 61b and ***61c*** shows you what the palatal build-up should look like. As we have discussed previously, they don't look like natural teeth.

FIGURE 60

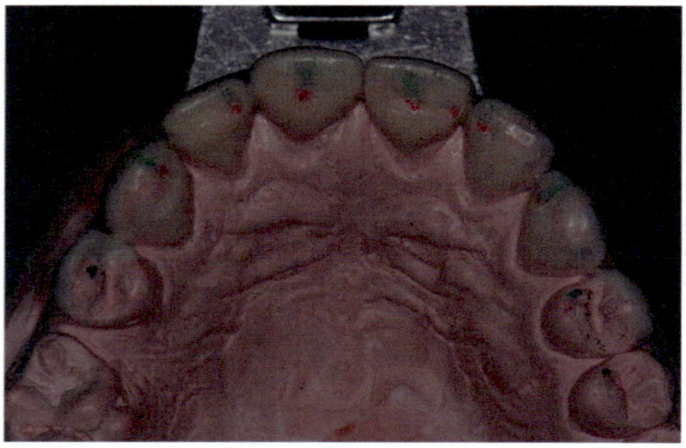

FIGURE 61a

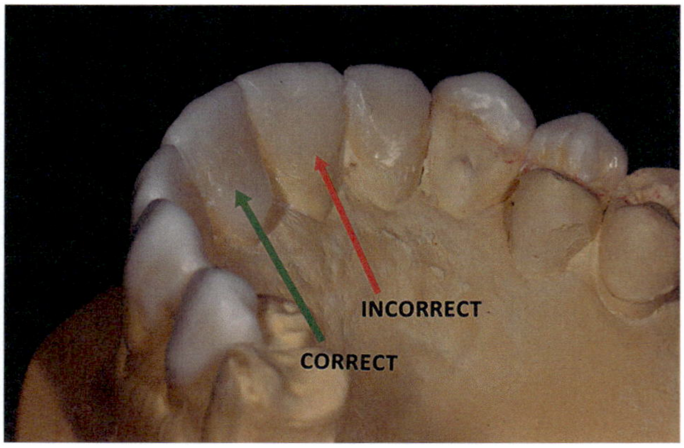

FIGURE 61b

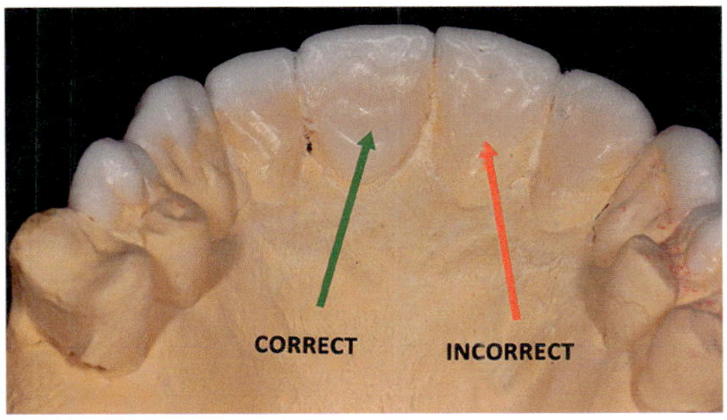

FIGURE 61c

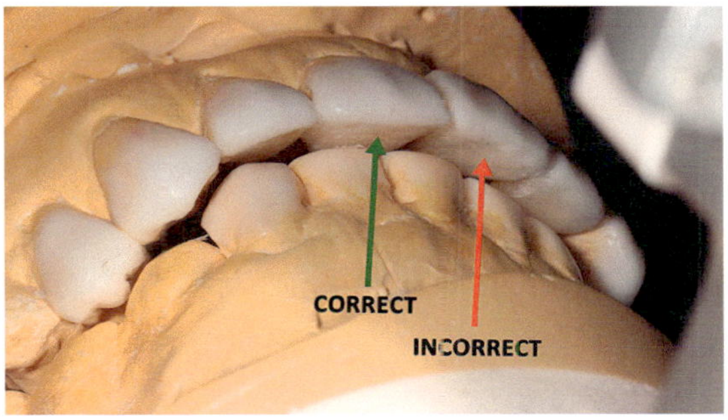

This is a biomechanical need, which is required in order to have that axial loading on the teeth.

Figure 62a and ***Figure 62b*** are the wax up I did for the patient in ***Figure 57.***

FIGURE 62a

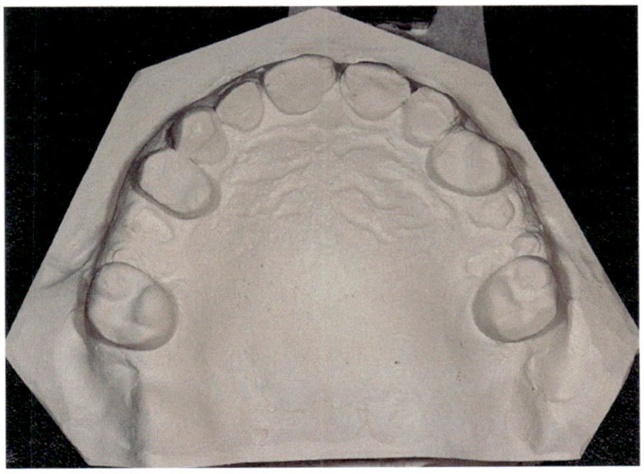

FIGURE 62b

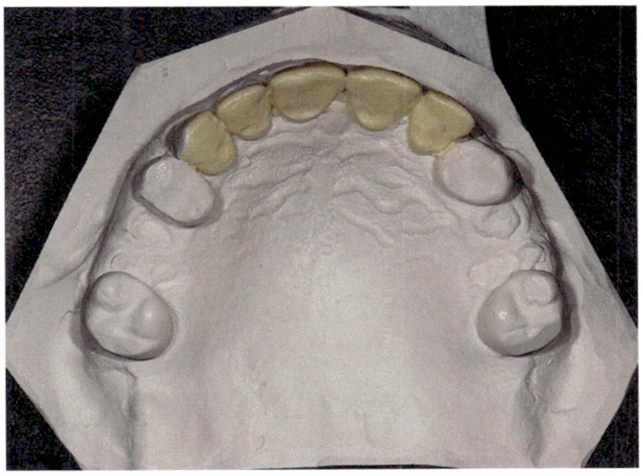

This is how it looks from the front in ***Figure 63***.

FIGURE 63a

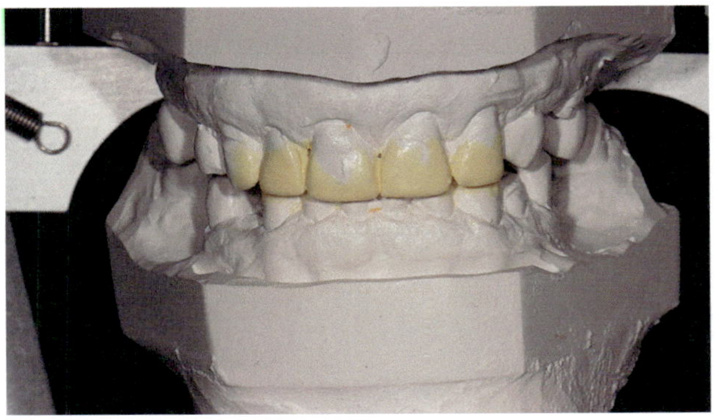

FIGURE 63b

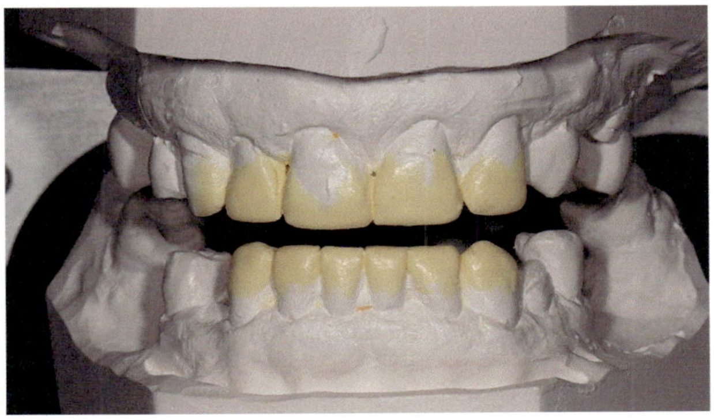

Appointment 4 - intraoral mock up

Once I have done the wax up, I am then going to do an intraoral mock-up using putty indices. I'll cut the putty and put a PTFE tape on the patient's interdental spaces if there are large undercuts.

Figure 64 shows the putty index to capture the wax up.

FIGURE 64

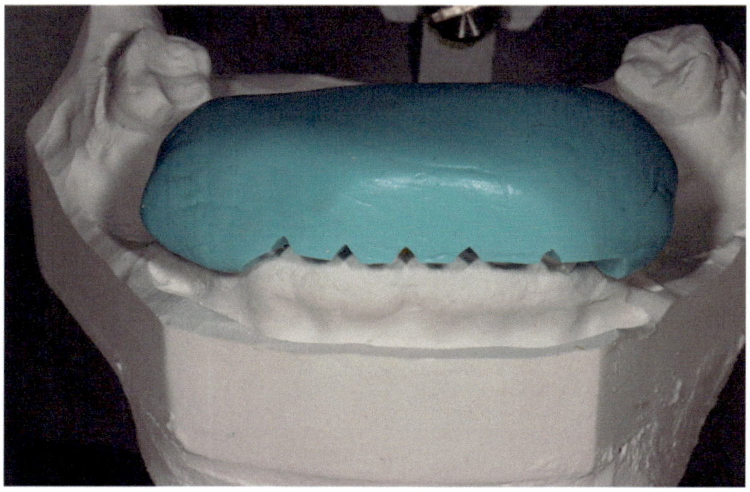

Then I would use temporary crown and bridge material in the putty and then in the patient's mouth to create a mock-up using the index from the diagnostic wax up.

Figure 65a shows indices and temporary crown and bridge material.

FIGURE 65a

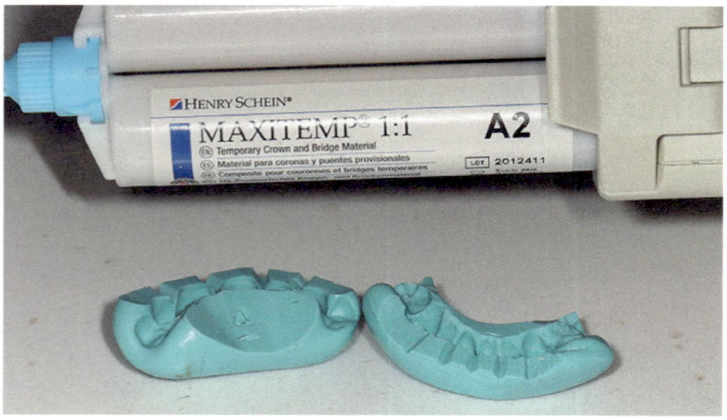

FIGURE 65b

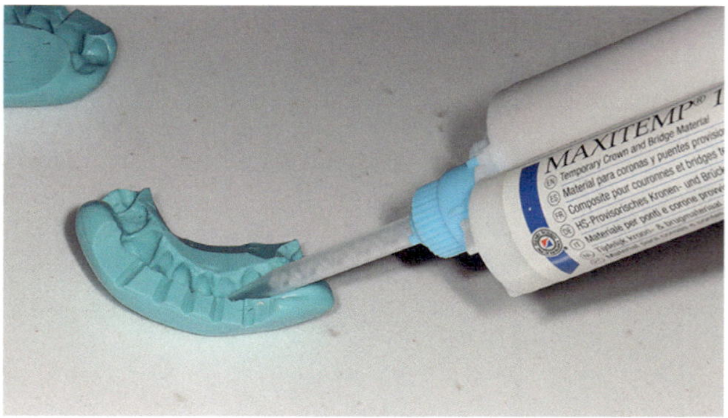

Figure 65b shows the insertion of temporary crown and bridge material into putty.

You can see a practical demonstration of how to use that diagnostic wax up and turn it into a mock-up in the patient's mouth in the online course called *Practical Guide to Full Mouth Reconstruction Book Course* which is free for the reader of this book. Please refer to the chapter entitled Links to Other Resources and scan the QR code to access it.

In the demonstration you will watch when you log into the course, I haven't created too many grooves and I haven't placed PTFE tape. But if you feel that there are large interdental spaces, then you can place PTFE tape in between the teeth to avoid material flowing into interdental areas.

If you haven't done it, you can still use a number 12 blade to carve the interdental spaces and remove any excess.

Assessing mock up

Once we have done the intraoral mock-up, we need to assess the aesthetic, phonetic, shade and occlusal factors.

Many times the shade is difficult to assess because it's acrylic. Sometimes you don't have different shades and you can't put in different characteristics.

You are going to check the occlusion to see if it is the same as your articulated model. If it's not the same and there is a small discrepancy then you can adjust the occlusion in the patient's mouth and retake the impressions to make duplicate models which you will use when taking indices for direct buildups.

However, if it's very far off from what you want then you need to really assess why you have got such a large discrepancy. You might even need to start again from scratch.

Before leaving the patient with the mock-up, make sure that the interdental spaces are clear and that they can clean properly between the teeth using interdental brushes. It will not be possible to floss as all the restorations will be connected and you need to inform the patient of this fact.

Once that's done I won't take the mock-up out - instead, I'll leave it with the patient to go home with. The patient needs to understand that even if things chip or break or get stained then I want them to try wearing it for at least a week.

Figure 66a shows the teeth straight after seating of the putty index with bisacry material.

FIGURE 66a

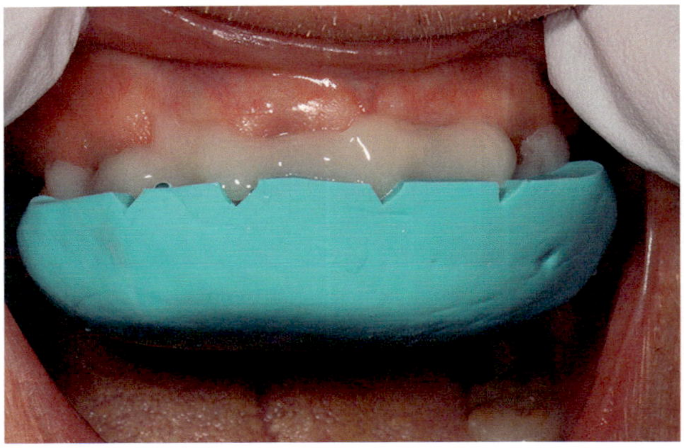

FIGURE 66b

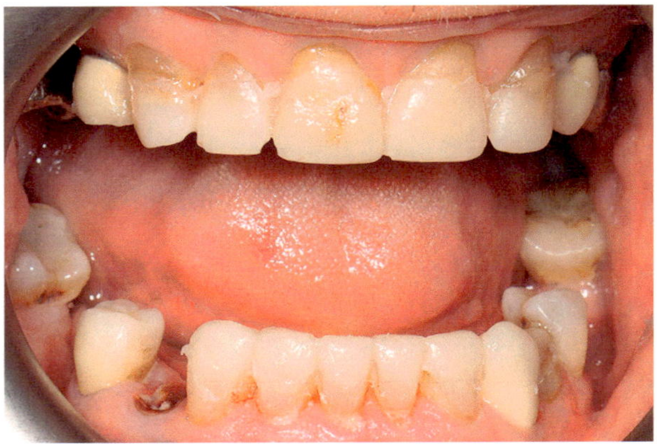

Figure 66b shows an open photo after cleaning the excess material.

Figure 66c shows teeth in occlusion.
Figure 66d shows confirming teeth are contacting in the same way as in the articulator.

FIGURE 66c

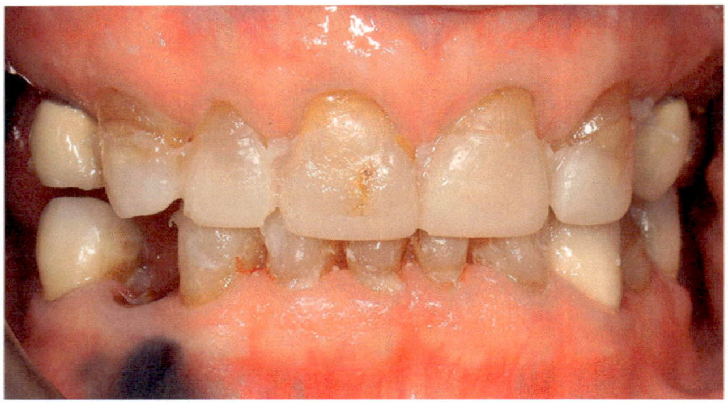

FIGURE 66d

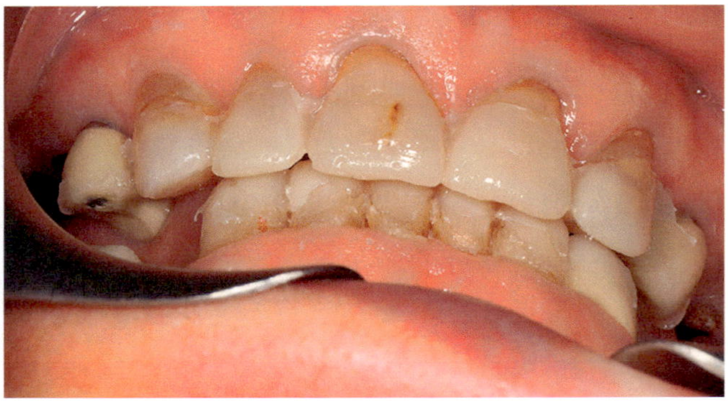

Figures 66a, 66b, 66c ,66d, 67a and ***67b*** are examples of the mock-up we did for a previous patient, and you can see how I'm assessing the contact points on the mock-up.

Figures 67a and ***67b*** show assessing occlusion.

FIGURE 67a

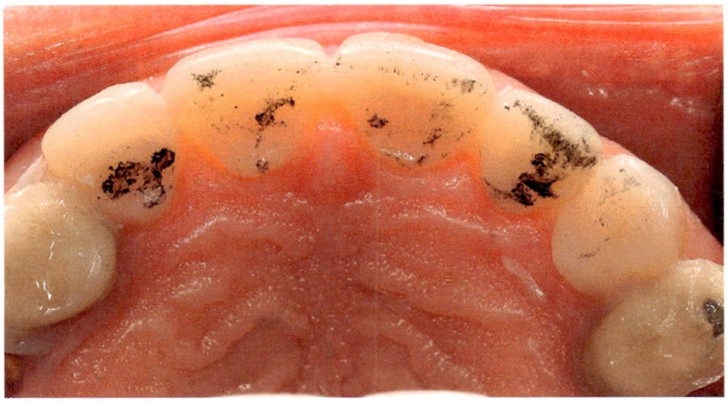

FIGURE 67b

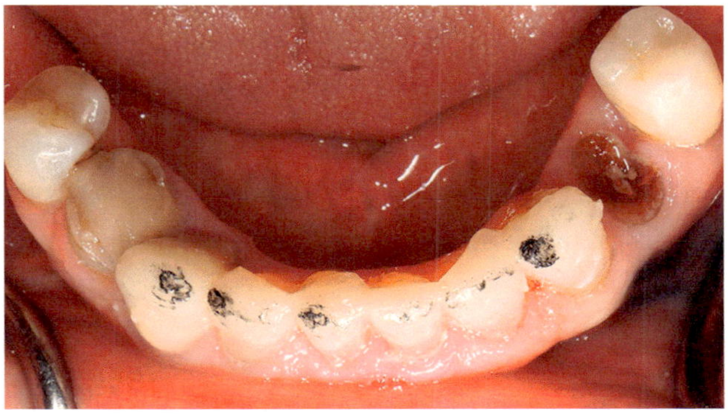

Appointment 5 - review mock-up after 1-2 weeks

When the patient comes back after a week or two, then we are going to check the occlusal contacts and the F, V, S, and TH sounds, whether the patient has got used to it or not. I'm also going to see if there has been any chipping in my restorations.

If there are any issues (like TMJ problems) then I won't proceed to the next step until I have found, verified and resolved the issue and checked again, and possibly (if it's needed) redo the mock-up. This is very important because until now we have not done anything that is irreversible.

Although we are doing a composite build-up, it's not completely reversible. As once you do some really nice composite bonding, it's impossible to remove 100% of the composite without damaging the tooth.

Therefore, you need to make sure you don't consider this to be a reversible treatment.

Appointment 6 - build-up for upper and lower canine to canine

Once we're happy with factors like the phonetics, the shape and the size, and the patient is happy with the occlusion, then we can move on to the next step, which is the build-up of the upper and lower canine to canine (front 6) teeth.

Why the anterior build-up first?

Many dentists have asked why they need to build the anterior teeth first as they might have been taught previously to build the posterior teeth first.

- I prefer doing the anterior teeth first because they are single-surface and easier to adjust.
- It's easier to change the OVD by adding a little bit or taking a little bit off.
- The condyles are seated very easily because all the work is being done away from the condyle. As we have discussed, there is likely to be less force as you go forward, which relaxes the jaw muscles which brings condyles into that CR position.

If you choose to treat the patient's posteriors first, then you risk locking them into their occlusion, which may reduce your ability to manage the anterior teeth because the posterior teeth come into contact first and shape of your anterior teeth will be then dictated by shape of the posterior teeth which may not be ideal.

Hence if you restore posterior teeth first then you cannot control the shape of the anterior teeth, which are much more important aesthetically than the posterior teeth. That's why you should build the anterior teeth first!

Methods of building anterior teeth:

- a direct build-up.
- an indirect build-up.
- a combination of a direct and indirect method.

Direct method

If you're doing a direct build-up you can do freehand, create putty indices or create clear indices using **Memosil** or **Exaclear (from GC).** You can also do injection moulding or a SmileFast UK technique.

Indirect method

If you're doing indirect, then you can use a composite, a porcelain or gold palatal backing, or a crown.

Direct/indirect method

If you're doing direct/indirect (semi-direct/sandwich) method then you will need to build-up the palatal surface and the incisal length using a composite. Once you've done all the reconstruction, you can then add veneers to the anterior teeth, keeping the palatal backing as it is.

This is a two-stage method, and many times I use it after my reconstruction is over as a purely cosmetic procedure.

Anterior build-up using a clear stent

Figure 68a and ***Figure 68b*** are examples of anterior wear. It's the same case as in ***Figure 66***.

FIGURE 68a

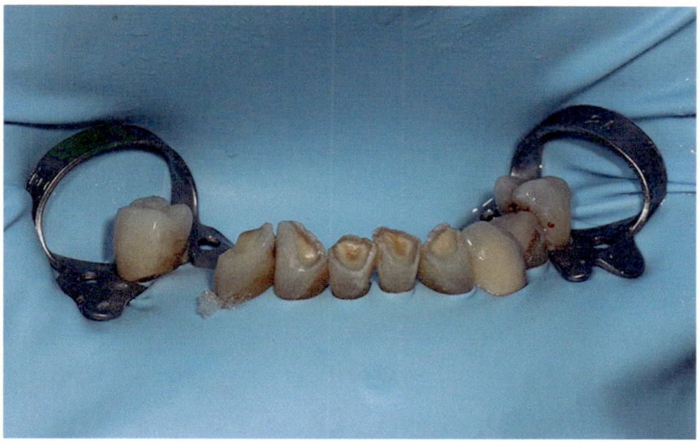

FIGURE 68b

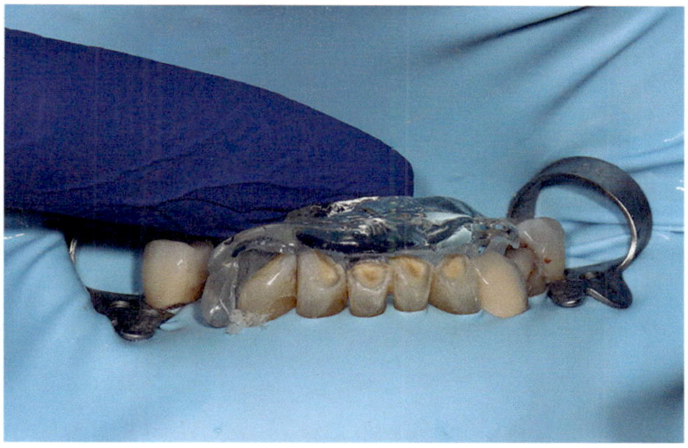

Figure 69 shows the result after the build-up.

FIGURE 69

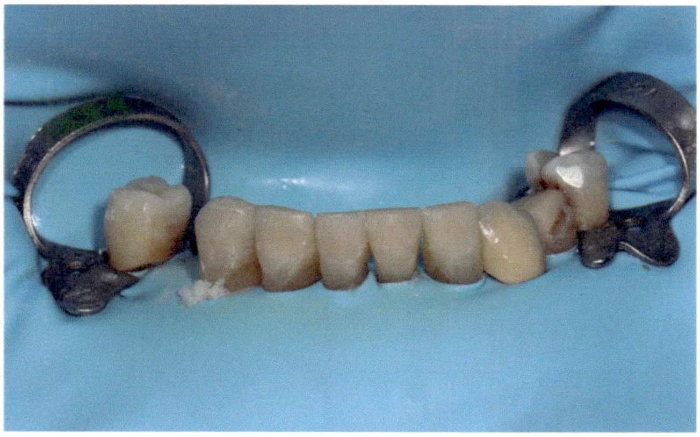

Checking occlusion

Once you've done the build-up you need to look at the guidance on the anterior teeth as shown in ***Figure 70*** (different case). You can see there are a lateral guidance on the canine and a protrusive guidance on the centrals and laterals.

FIGURE 70

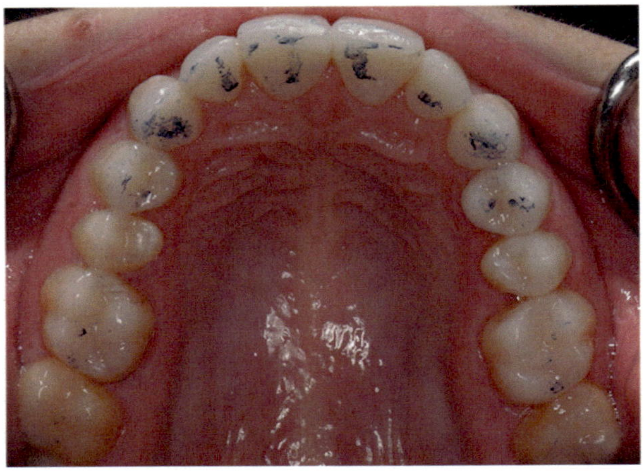

Stabilising posteriors

Once we build the front teeth, we need to stabilise the posterior teeth because we're not going to restore them on the same day. You don't want to leave the patient in the same position, otherwise the condylar resetting might happen, you may end up losing the space, or the patient might not get used to it. Therefore, you will want to place something on the posterior teeth just to stabilise the occlusion.

Temporarisation strategies

If you're doing direct adhesive composite restoration, then you can build the anterior teeth using composite and temporise the posterior teeth using a GIC stop. Therefore, you literally place the GIC on each tooth, making sure you take the rubber dam out first, and then you put the GIC on the lower teeth or just the upper teeth and ask the patient to close. Apply Vaseline petroleum jelly on the opposite side to avoid GIC sticking to the opposite teeth when the patient closes their mouth. This will make sure the patient contacts the front teeth and the posterior teeth and GIC stop will adjust accordingly.

I will do a GIC stop per tooth and place them right in the middle of the occlusal surface, making sure they stay within the marginal ridges.

Do not extend GIC stops to the marginal ridges, because when you take new impressions for a second wax up, your technician needs to know the outline of the tooth. So, you're going to place the GIC in the middle of the occlusal surface.

Figure 71a is an example showing how to place GIC stops. You can see what the GIC stops look like. They are not extending and are not connected, as they are all separate stops. In ***Figure 71b*** you can see that when the patient has come back for the bonding for posterior, I will remove GIC on the alternate teeth and use my indices to build those teeth using stamp technique. GIC stops removed from LL6 and LL4 before building those two teeth. GIC stops on the LL5 and LL7 were kept to provide support for the indices. Once those two teeth were built, gic stops were removed from LL5 and LL7 to build those teeth.

Figure 71a shows GIC stops without covering marginal ridges.

FIGURE 71a

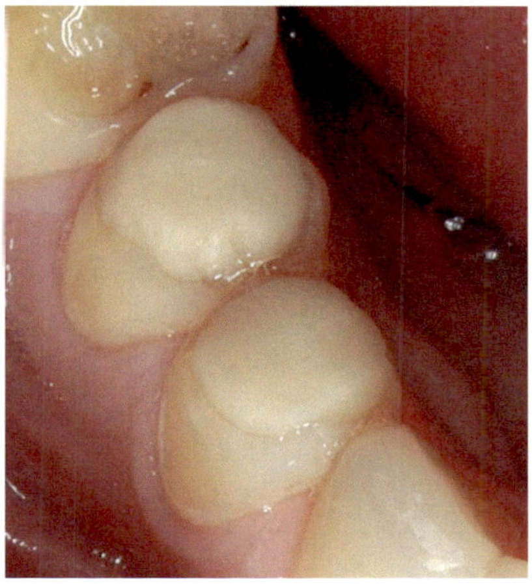

FIGURE 71b

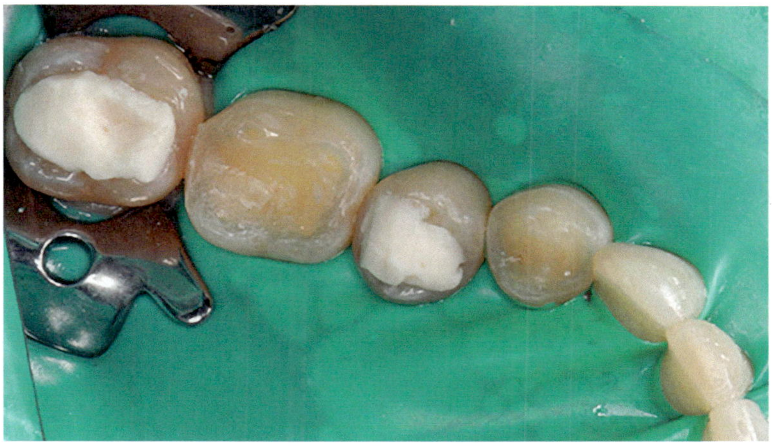

An alternative strategy is to use an index from the wax up and use temporary crown and bridge material to shrink fit the acrylic as you would do for your temporary crown or onlays.

In ***Figure 72a*** and ***72b,*** this is what you would usually see on the top photos when you've done the anterior build-ups. You will see that the posterior teeth are not in contact, so you can put in some GIC stops to stabilise the bite. ***Figure 72c*** and ***72d*** shows photos after build ups.

FIGURE 72a

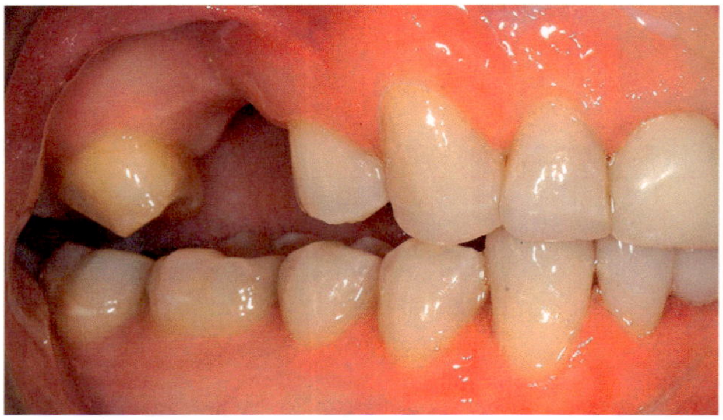

FIGURE 72b

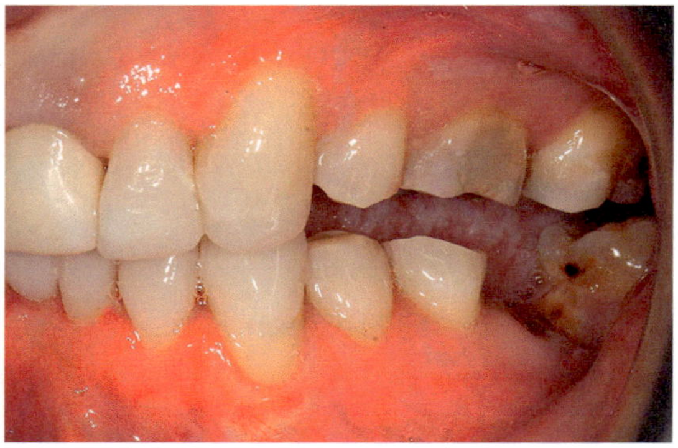

FIGURE 72c

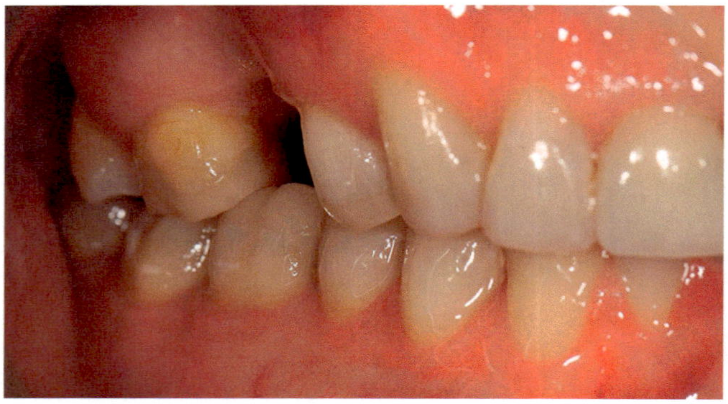

FIGURE 72d

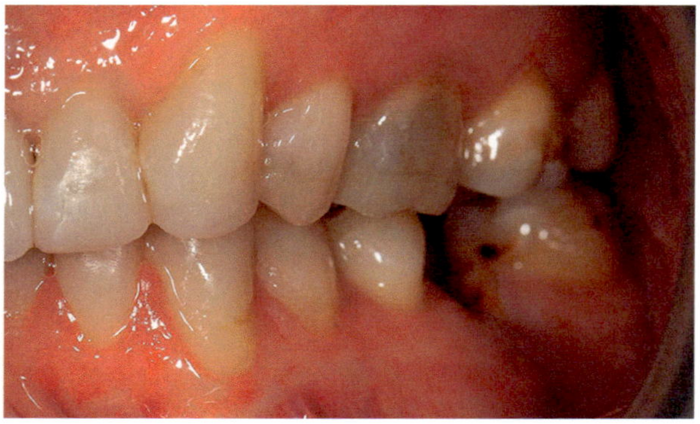

Appointment 7 - review + second wax up (once anterior restorations are stable)

So let's say we've done an anterior build-up and put some GIC stops on the posterior teeth. The next thing you need to do is a secondary wax up because you may have inevitably adjusted the anterior teeth, polishing and changing the occlusion a little bit. To get a more accurate result you need to re-take the impression of the upper and lower teeth and re-mount the model in ICP (as your new ICP = CO).

You may need to place some bite registration material on the posterior if the teeth are not contacting properly. Then you can just mount the model (like in ICP) and do the wax up.

Alternative tooth wax up for posterior teeth (premolar to molar)

In these two wax ups (shown in ***Figure 73a*** and ***Figure 73b)*** you're going to focus on where the alternative teeth are waxed-up first. First you will wax up alternative teeth like in Figure 73a and then, you'll duplicate the model and then continue with the wax up like in ***Figure 73b***.

You can see the build-up of the rest of the teeth. Here, we were not restoring third molars and hence we haven't waxed up those teeth.

FIGURE 73a

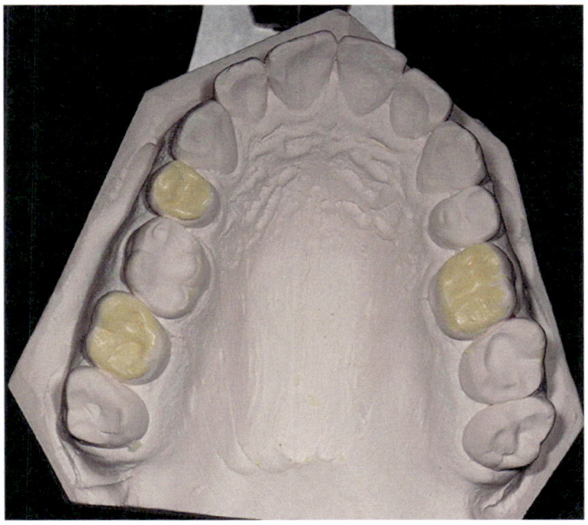

FIGURE 73b

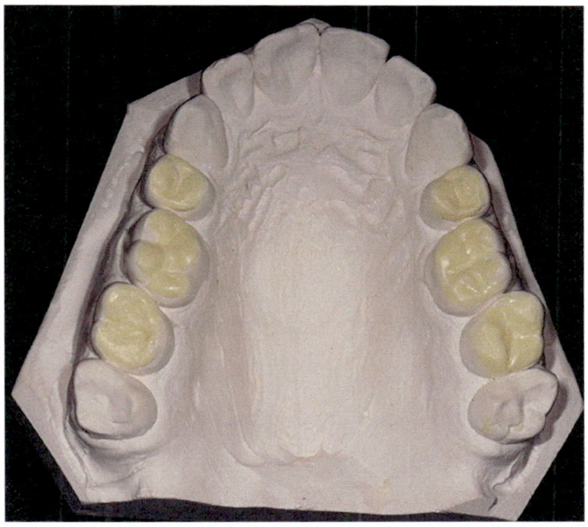

On the lower teeth in ***Figure 74a***, also shows alternative teeth wax up. It does not matter if you do one tooth first or the other, as far as waxed up teeth have teeth without wax on either side. The reason you are doing the alternative tooth is because you can take the indices of the alternative wax model first **(*Figure 73a*** and ***Figure 74a***), build those teeth with the composite, and then take the indices of the fully waxed up model **(*Figure 73b*** and ***Figure 74b***) and build the remaining teeth. That will make sure that your indices are stable when you are using stamp technique and excess is less.

FIGURE 74a

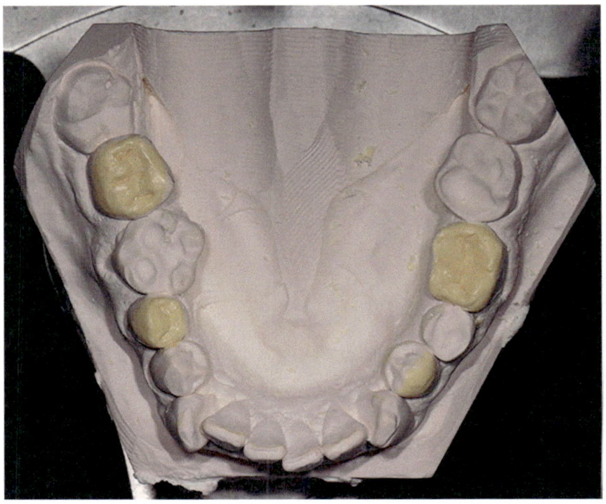

FIGURE 74b

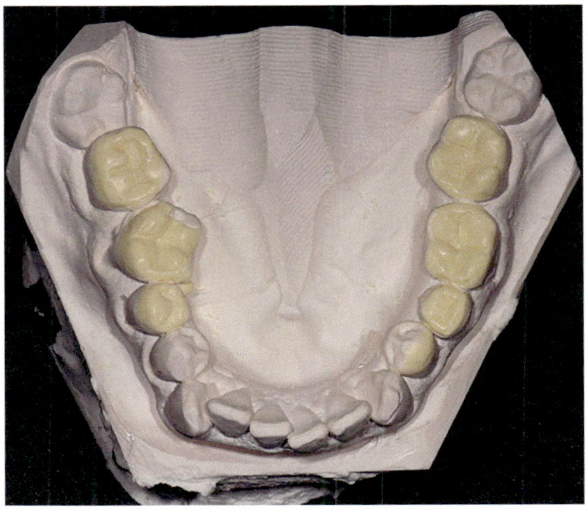

If you have waxed up all the teeth and are now trying to stabilise the indices, then it will not be stable. Your composite, if you're using the stamp method or stamp technique, will flow into the other tooth and leave you with connected teeth.

Therefore, it's very important that you ask the technician to do an alternative teeth wax up. It is simpler if you are doing digital wax up as you can just undo the wax up easily and print model with alternative tooth wax up.

Appointment 8 – posterior build-up

Now we are doing a posterior build-up. This can be done via a direct restoration or indirect restoration.

Direct restoration:

If you're doing a direct then you can use a stamp method, which is my favourite as it's quick and easy, especially when you're doing something direct. Usually, you would do something direct when the build-up is around 2 mm or less, which is when the step method would work.

You can use putty indices, but it's a bit trickier for the posterior teeth. You can use a direct free hand to build up, but this is guesswork and that becomes a bit trickier.

Indirect restorations:

With regards to indirect, you can do onlays or crowns using different materials. If I'm doing an indirect restoration then I make sure that I have the provisionals in place first before I move on to definitive restorations.

You can do a veneer-lays for posterior premolars or molars (mainly premolars) where you have a veneer on the buccal and then veneers extending on the occlusal surface. This is because when you raise the OVD and have occlusal space to fill, you can extend your veneer on the occlusal surface and the patient can close on it.

As discussed before, you can do one arch at a time or one side at a time. If you are doing one arch at a time them you need to start with the lower arch to make sure you maintain a flat Curve of Spee and aesthetics of lower teeth. If you are doing one side at a time then you can decide whichever side you would like to do first. If you are doing one side at a time then it gives you much more control. However, you need to make sure that your arch, once you do the final restoration, is in line with the cosmetic appearance or the smile (if you're doing one side at a time) as it's easy for you to lose that sense of perception and one side can become smaller or longer than the other side.

Appointment 9 - build another side (left upper and lower posteriors) or build another arch

Once you have completed one arch at a time or one side at a time then you need to complete the other side or other arch.

Figure 75a shows the lower right posterior wear, whereas the photo in ***Figure 75b*** is taken after the direct composite restoration using the stamp technique. ***Figure 75c*** shows the upper right posterior wear. ***Figure 75d*** shows the teeth after direct composite restoration using stamp technique.

FIGURE 75a

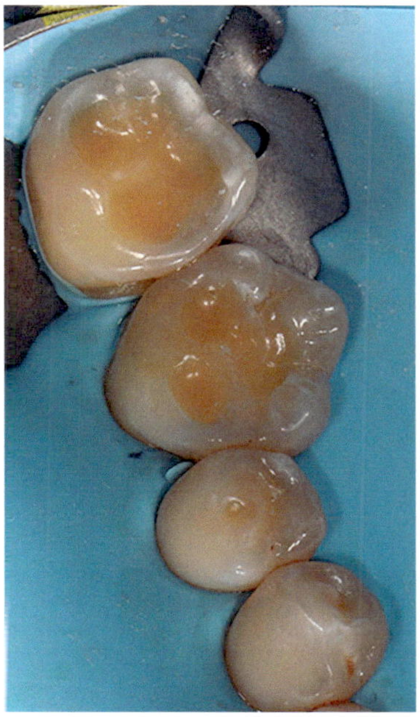

FIGURE 75b

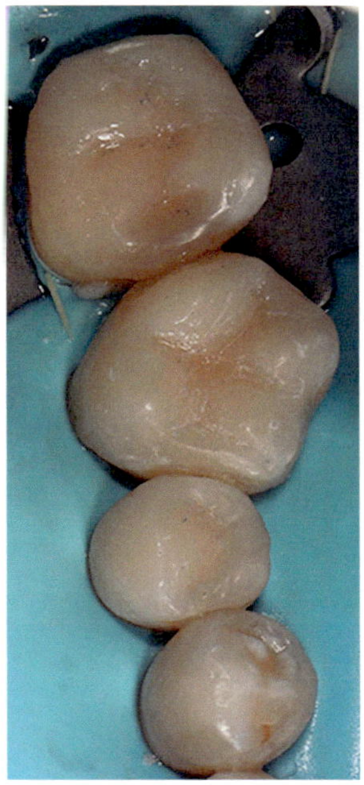

FIGURE 75c

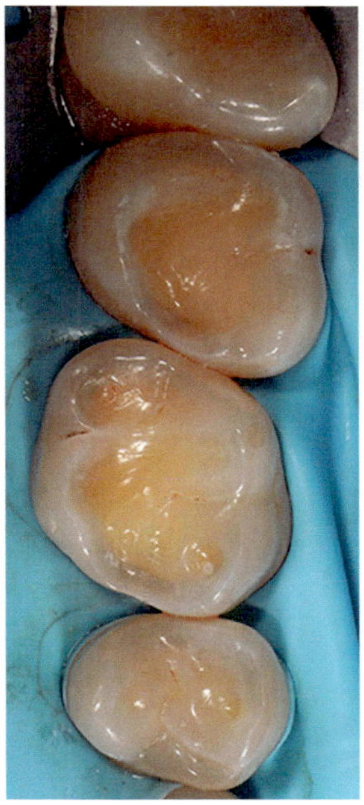

FIGURE 75d

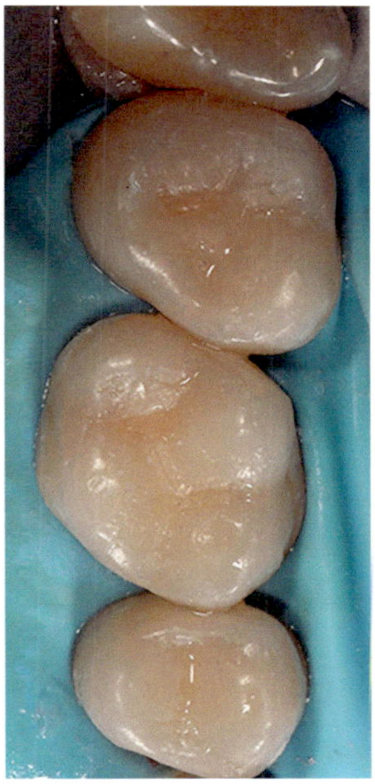

During appointment 9, you swap to the other side if you've done one side.

Figure 76a shows lower left posterior wear, and ***Figure 76b*** shows the tooth after completion of direct restoration using stamp technique.

FIGURE 76a

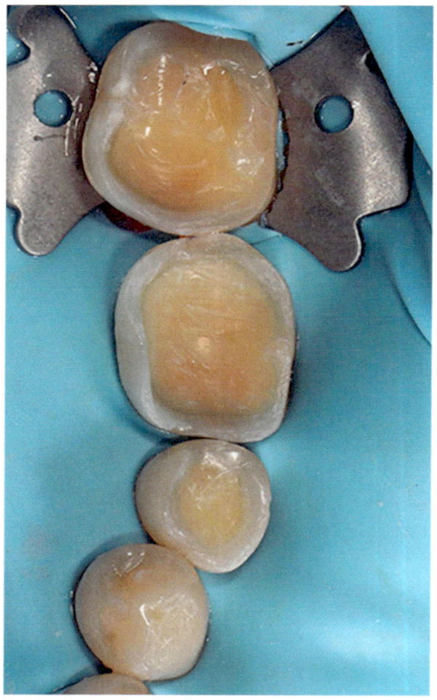

FIGURE 76b

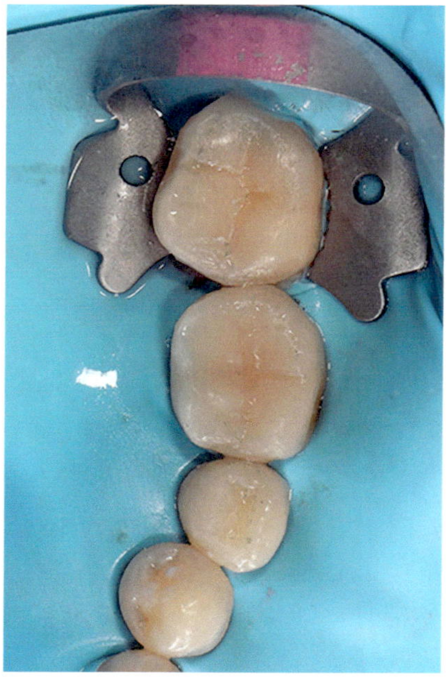

Figure 77a shows upper left posterior wear, ***Figure 77b*** shows after completion of direct restoration using stamp technique.

FIGURE 77a

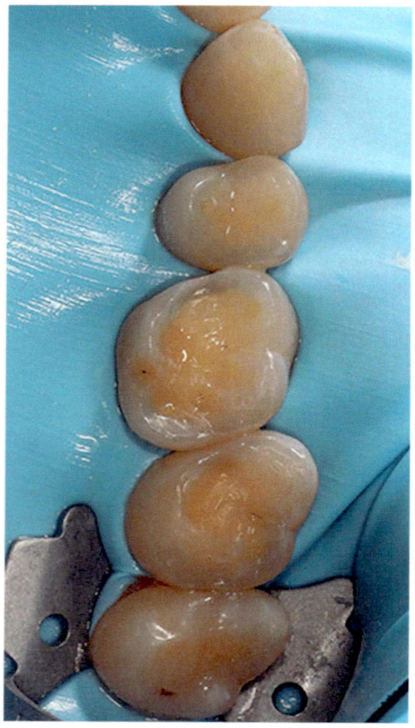

FIGURE 77b

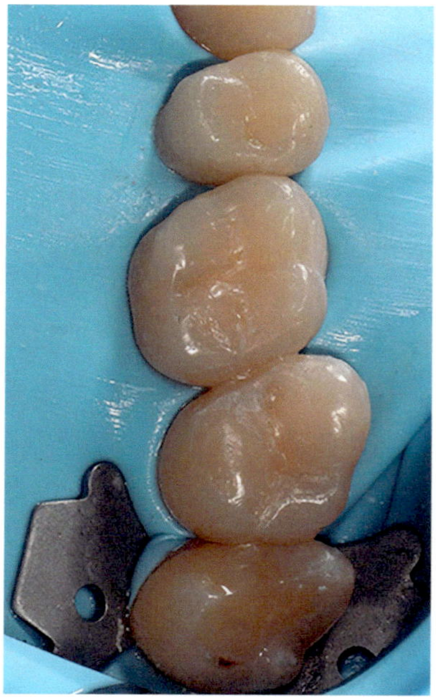

Appointment 10 - review + record for the Michigan splint

Once you've done all that, check and refine the occlusion and once you're happy with it review the process with a couple of review appointments.

Appointment 11 – fit the Michigan splint

Once you're happy then you're going to make the Michigan Splint (***Figure 78***), taking the records for it and fitting it. As discussed before, you may choose to give the patient a soft night guard or dual arch B splint.

FIGURE 78

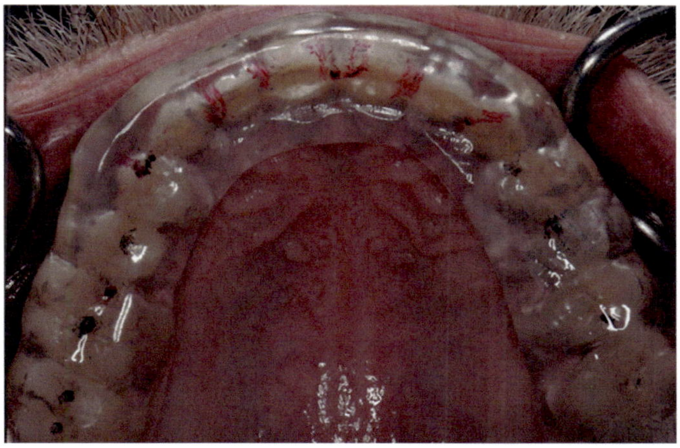

Appointment 12 - review and maintenance

Now you need to place your patient on a maintenance regime, which means regular hygiene appointments and using high fluoride toothpaste if they need it.

This is alongside additional yearly maintenance for polishing, composite repair, or maintenance of the implant prosthesis.

Minimally invasive reconstruction

Now you can hopefully see how to plan and how to start. *Always* start with treatment planning.

Figure 79a shows a front view of tooth surface loss (TSL). ***Figure 79b*** shows teeth in occlusion.

FIGURE 79a

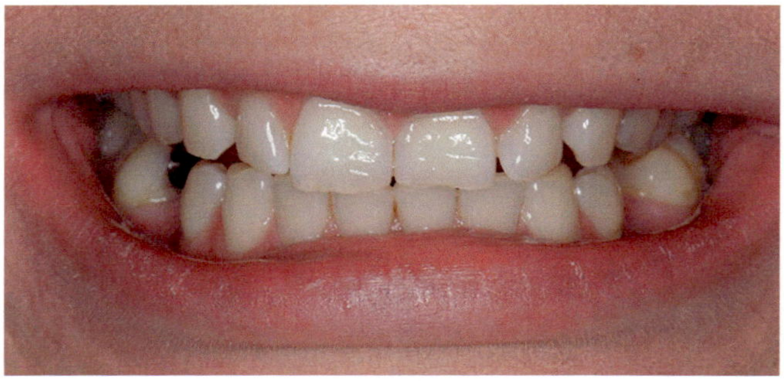

FIGURE 79b

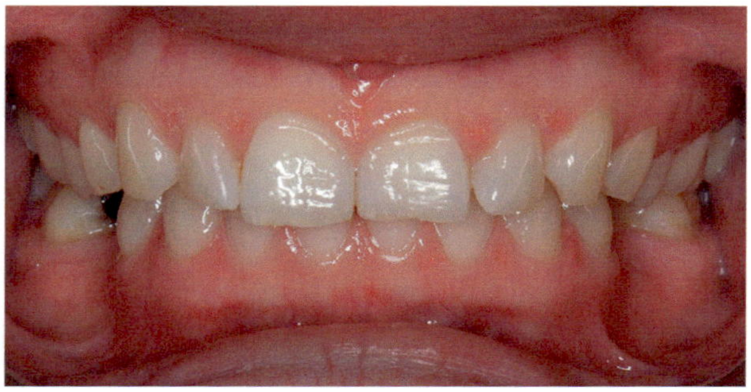

Figure 79c shows the upper arch showing moderate wear and ***Figure 79d*** shows lower arch showing mild wear.

FIGURE 79c

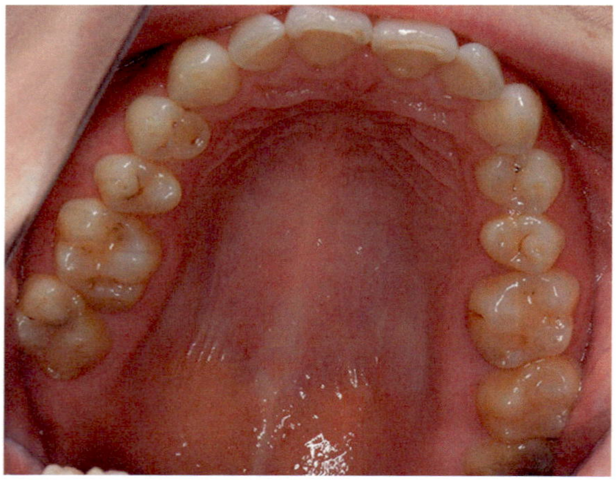

FIGURE 79d

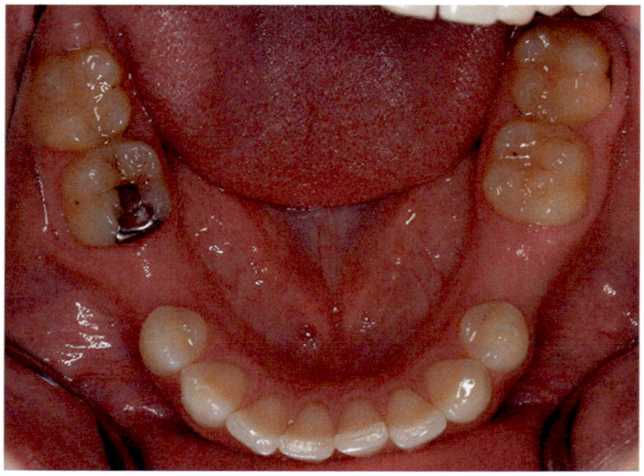

Treatment flow for adhesive direct full mouth reconstructions

Step 1: Treatment planning

- Comprehensive assessment.
- Impression and records.

- Mounting models in CR/CO or ICP (which is very rare as usually we mount a model in CR or CO).
- Diagnostic wax up.
- Trying out the mock-up of that diagnostic wax up.

Step 2: Anterior build-ups

- Upper and lower anterior definitive restoration.
- Stabilisation of the posterior teeth.

Step 3: Posterior build-ups and maintenance

- Restoring posterior teeth (one side at a time or one arch at a time).
- Maintaining and protecting your restorations.
- Providing the patient with some maintenance options.

Think!

You will need to take CR records if you're doing a diagnostic wax up.

In this case because there's minor to moderate tooth surface loss, a direct restoration was needed.

Again, the steps you're going to follow are: comprehensive assessment, records, mounting, wax up, mock-up, upper and lower anterior restoration, stabilising the posterior, the posterior restoration, and protection and maintenance.

Once you have finished, you'll have a predictable result, one which allows you to see even contacts and guidance in the mouth and the restoration of the patient's upper and lower dentition.

Figure 80a shows a smile photo after a finished anterior result, ***Figure 80b*** shows the retracted view, ***Figure 80c*** shows the occlusal view of maxillary teeth and ***Figure 80d*** shows the occlusal view of mandibular teeth as a completion of the treatment.

FIGURE 80a

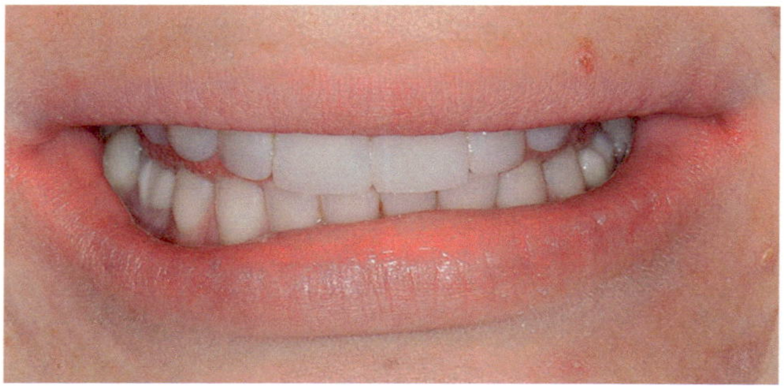

FIGURE 80b

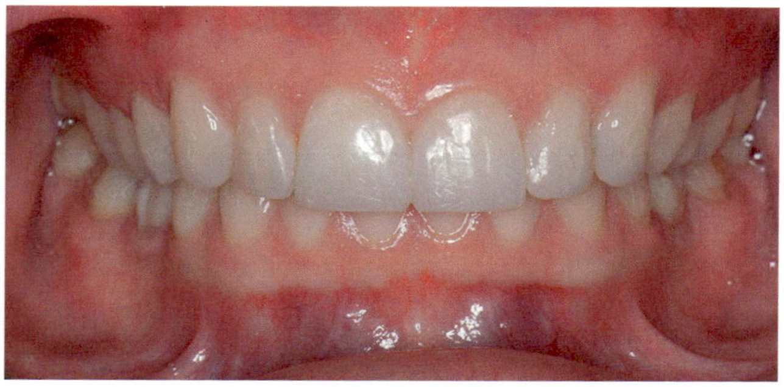

FIGURE 80c

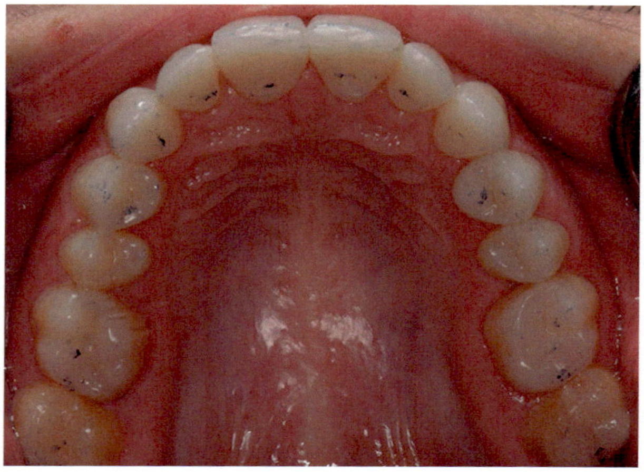

FIGURE 80d

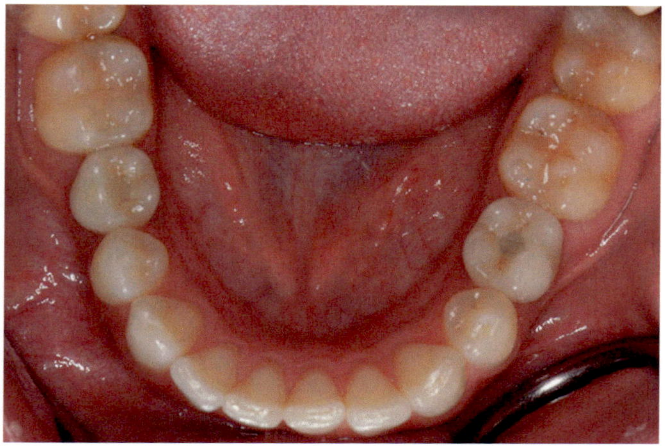

I hope this has given you a sense of what the step-by-step process involves. If anything is unclear, then it's advisable to read the chapter again as this is a crucial aspect of full mouth reconstruction. Once you've followed all the steps, the process will become easier and most of your patients for direct adhesive cases will fit into this pattern.

Let's say you're dealing with a removable prosthodontic, such as a denture. You're going to build all the teeth up first and then provide the patient with the denture.

However, if you're doing indirect restorations like crowns or onlays, then you can provide rest seats on those teeth for your chrome denture in which case you need to plan the denture and the indirect restorations together with your technicians.

So there are lots of different ways you can plan the treatment. Yet I want you to learn one way and start with the simple cases, getting the fundamentals and learning the basics of full mouth reconstruction before doing anything more complex.

2.5 Diagnostic Wax Up

In this chapter we will discuss the subject of diagnostic wax up.

Why diagnostic wax up?

So let's look at the advantages of diagnostic wax up and why I would recommend you do it whenever you're doing full mouth reconstruction.

- Diagnostic wax up helps you in **visualising the endpoint**, the shape and the contour of your restorations.
- It also assesses and **manages the patient's expectations** through a physical mockup which shows them what is realistic. While you're taking indices from the diagnostic wax up and placing this into the patient's mouth and assessing this, then you will understand what the patient's expectations are versus what can be achieved. Many times, even if you're doing digital analysis and showing the patient photographs, they cannot feel the final result. However, when you transfer that mock-up into the patient's mouth your patient can envision the end goal. This really **helps with communication** because if the patient does not like the mock up then you can go back to the drawing board and start asking questions again before proceeding.
- Diagnostic wax up is done before you have done any irreversible damage in most cases. So, if the patient doesn't like it you can go back to the drawing board and change your wax up until your patient is happy with it. I would not recommend proceeding with treatment until your patient is completely satisfied with the wax up.
- Wax up also helps you in **assessing planned occlusion.** You can change possible occlusion after you've done the mock-up, so this helps you in planning the future occlusion of your restoration.
- Sometimes when you are restoring teeth you are not sure whether the spaces are big enough, or small enough, for you to give your patient the right shape. Again this is a situation where diagnostic wax up, digital or analogue diagnostic wax up will help you in **planning the case**. If you are not sure about the shape or your patient cannot visualise how it will look then diagnostic wax up is very helpful.

- Once you have a diagnostic wax up, which is approved by the patient, you can **make indices** and you can use this as a reduction guide when you are doing your preparation. By doing this you will make sure that you are neither over- nor underreducing the tooth when you're doing preparation.
- It can also help you in **fabricating provisional restorations**. I always take indices from my diagnostic wax up to make the first set of provisional restorations.

So when you're doing diagnostic wax up what are you aiming for?

Whenever I am doing a diagnostic wax up, or I am asking the technician to carry out a diagnostic wax up, then I am looking for occlusal stability with the maximum aesthetic outcome.

What is occlusal stability and why do we want occlusal stability in our restorations?

- Occlusal stability helps you in **reducing ongoing wear** in the patient's teeth. You are giving the patient the freedom to move their jaw around without locking their jaw or creating steep guidance.
- It reduces wear; it doesn't increase the mobility of the teeth and **mitigates the trauma from occlusion**.
- It ensures that the **restorations are durable.**
- It makes sure that this **TMJ is symptom free**.

How can we achieve occlusal stability?

- We achieve occlusal stability by giving the patient multiple and even contacts in ICP after the completion of the treatment.
- Make sure that the forces are axially directed for posterior teeth and if you are doing DAHL technique then, as we discussed, forces are axially directed for the anterior teeth as well.
- In ICP anterior teeth have a very light contact and heavy contact on posterior teeth. There is an immediate disclusion of the posterior teeth by creating shallow guidance from the anterior teeth. This way posterior teeth protects anterior during heavy axial loading and anterior teeth protects posterior teeth during destructive lateral forces. This is called ***mutually protected occlusion***.

Anterior teeth

Here we are asking our technician to fabricate the anterior teeth. Make sure you have axial loading even for anterior teeth as discussed before, especially when you are doing DAHL and the shallow guidance with immediate disclusion of the posterior teeth with jaw movement.

Again in this ***Figure 81*** where we discussed palatal ramp, when we are doing DAHL or even if doing full mouth reconstruction we want the anterior teeth to be axially loaded.

FIGURE 81

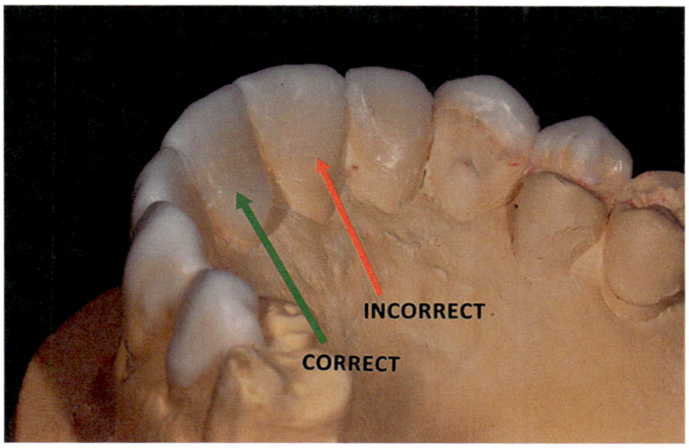

You can see the differences between the right upper central which is the correct one and the left central which is incorrect one in ***Figure 81***, ***Figure 82*** and ***Figure 83***.

FIGURE 82

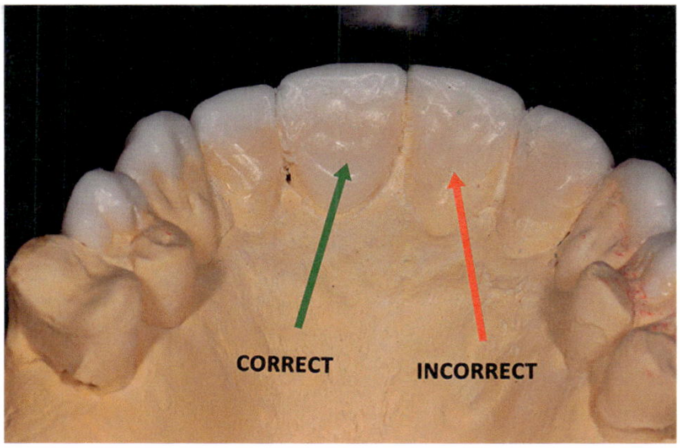

FIGURE 83

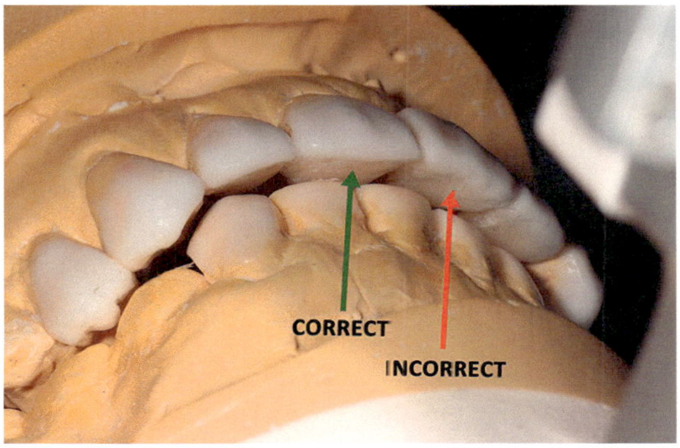

Many times technicians wax up teeth like the left central incisor because the normal shape of the teeth is like that. However, what we are trying to create on the right central is a more biomechanical surface of the tooth, where the forces are axially loaded. This is not very natural but it does make sure that your restorations are stable and gives you that occlusal stability.

Posterior teeth

With regards to posterior teeth we want again forces to be directed axially. We can do that by creating tripodisation. We have discussed that sometimes tripodisation is very difficult and in those cases we are using both flat surface and point contact from the opposite teeth as shown in ***Figure 84.***

FIGURE 84

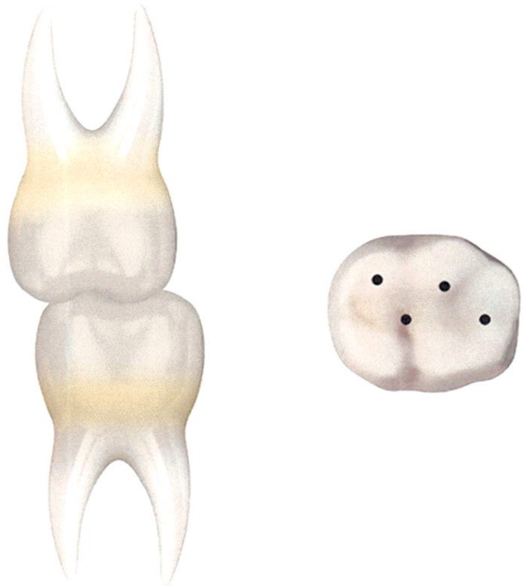

We want a ridge to fossa relationship rather than cusp to marginal ridge relationship.

Let's look at some practical demonstrations on how to do diagnostic wax up. Please enrol into my free online Practical Guide to Full mouth reconstruction book course to view the demonstration. Once again you can find it here:

When you use coupon code 'fmrbook' the course will be free for you.

As usual, if you are having issues accessing the link by using the QR code, then make sure to contact me at https://drdevangpatel.com/contact/.

I am personally fond of doing wax up and I quite frequently do my own diagnostic wax ups, especially for adhesive cases where I'm going to do direct composite buildups.

If I am doing indirect restoration then I am going to ask my technician to do the wax up. This is because I need to know their understanding of the shapes, as ultimately they are going to make the veneers, crowns or onlay and I need to make sure that their understanding of the shape is exactly the same as my understanding of the shape and occlusion. So if you're asking your technician to do the wax up, and then make sure that you are asking them to send the models back with an articulator so then you can assess the wax up properly.

There is no point in having a study model with wax up without an articulator because you cannot assess the wax up properly.

As you may have realised that diagnostic wax up is a very important part of the full mouth reconstruction and whether you do this digitally or via analogue rout, it cannot be missed.

Once you have carried out the diagnostic wax up and have done a mock up which is approved by your patient then you can move on to the **step 2** which is anterior build up.

CHAPTER 3

Step 2: Anterior Reconstruction

3.1 The Art of Bonding

In this section we are going to discuss the art of bonding. You need to understand bonding, especially when you're doing direct full mouth reconstruction.

Key aspect of art of bonding

In order to understand bonding, you need to understand four main areas related to bonding which are **isolation, bonding agents, immediate dentin sealing and bonding protocol.**

Isolation

- Isolating the tooth at the time of the bonding procedure is very important, to avoid any contamination from the saliva but also to give you as much time as you need, without stress. If you were to isolate a tooth without a rubber dam, you can't expect your patient to keep their tongue still forever. If the patient's tongue is moving around the mouth, saliva will also be distributed around the mouth. This can potentially contaminate the area when you are bonding; it will make the procedure stressful for you and give you an incentive to rush. All this would mean your work would not be your best. A rubber dam is the absolute best practice.
- If a rubber dam is not practical because there is a deep margin on the tooth and the margins are gingival, then you should consider doing deep marginal elevation.

Figure 85a is an example where I have isolated the anterior and one posterior quadrant. You can see in ***Figure 85b*** that even though I'm restoring anterior canine to canine, I am isolating significantly further back.

FIGURE 85a

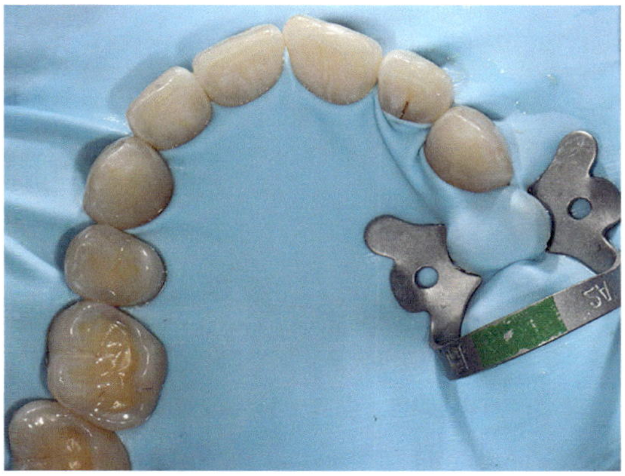

FIGURE 85b

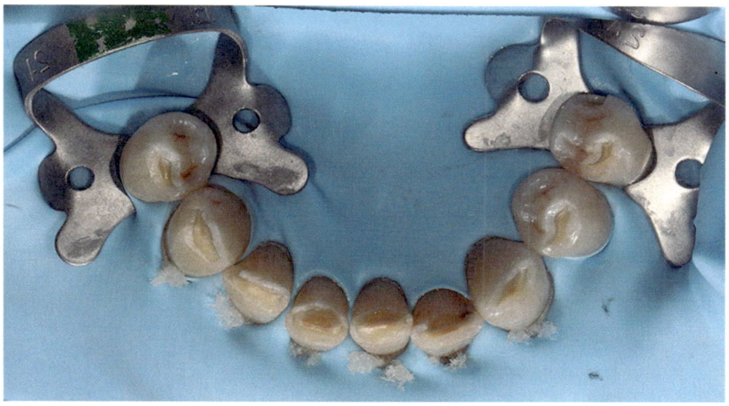

I could go not further back than the premolar in ***Figure 85b*** because there were no teeth behind those two teeth. Otherwise, if there is a molar I would go right up to the second or first molar at least to isolate those teeth. The idea is to isolate as much wider area as possible to allow ample access.

Figure 86 is an example of deep caries. We restored that tooth by doing deep margin elevation followed by an onlay ***(Figure 87)***.

FIGURE 86

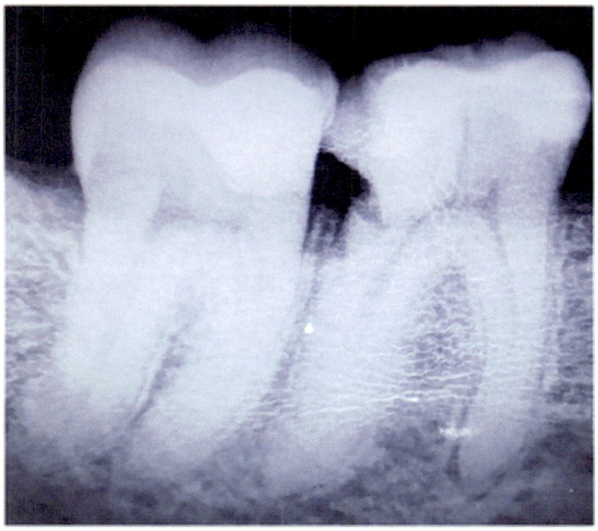

FIGURE 87

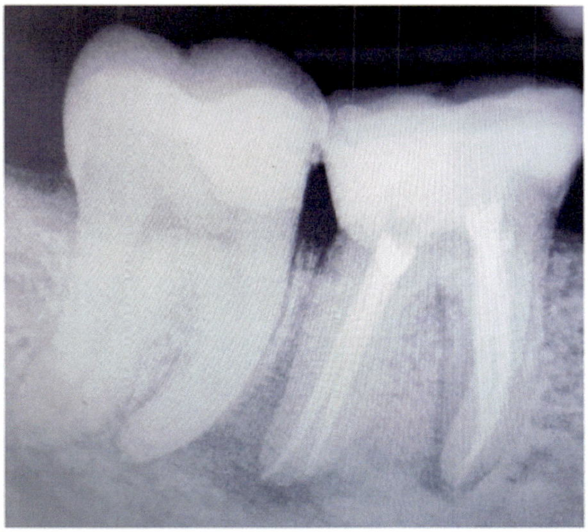

Bonding agents

- Since the invention of bonding agent dental treatment has become much more conservative. We have been able to save much more tooth tissue. In the old days when the bonding agents weren't very good, the only way to protect teeth was to crown them and we all know crowning teeth destroys a lot of enamel.

The adhesive systems are composed of a monomer with both hydrophilic group and hydrophobic group. It is very important because teeth are composed of enamel, dentin and pulp. Out of these, we can only bond to enamel and dentine. But both of them have different characteristics.

Hydrophilic part helps with bonding to dentine as dentine is wet due to water content and the hydrophobic part helps bonding with resin which does not like water. This way we can get predictable bonding with dentine. As we know bonding to enamel is very predictable and hence it is not an issue in general.

As you can see from this table they are completely different. Enamel is made up of mainly inorganic material whereas dentine has a lot more organic phase and water than enamel.

Table 5:

Components	Enamel	Dentine
Inorganic phase (mainly hydroxyapatite) (%)	94-96	50-70
Calcium phosphate ratio	1.64	1.56
Organic phase (mainly collagen) (%)	4-5	20-30
Water (%)	1-4	10-20

And now what we are doing is we are trying to bond enamel and dentine together in one procedure. Our composite must bond to enamel and dentin at the same time and that's where the challenge occurs.

That's not the only issue. The other issue is the smear layer.

Smear layer removal – total etch or self-etch

Smear layer happens when you are cutting a tooth, removing decay. The debris sometimes gets embedded into the dentine and most of the new dentin agents or bonding agents are concentrating on how to remove the smear layer because we know from the studies that the smear layer blocks the resin tags. Because of this we cannot get hybrid layers to the standard we want.

In order to get the high standard hybrid layer connection between your bonding agent and dentine, you will want to remove that smear layer. There are different ways to remove the smear layer, I will outline two of what are considered the best practice methods.

- First using total etch which means you etch enamel and dentine at the same time and clean everything up, removing the smear layer completely.
- Second, self-etch where you're not really etching dentine separately but you're using a primer which includes the etching ability and it basically dissolves the smear layer or penetrates through the smear layer to create that hybrid layer and it supposedly helps in reducing sensitivity.

Classification of bonding agents by generation

Table 6:

Generations	Number of Steps	Surface Pre-Treatment	Components
1st	2	Enamel etch	2
2nd	2	Enamel etch	2
3rd	3	Dentine conditioning	2-3
4th	3	Total etch	3
5th	2	Total etch	2
6th	1	Self-etch adhesive	2
7th	1	Self-etch adhesive	1
8th	1	Self-etch adhesive	1

There are eight generations of bonding agents and they all have different uses and were invented for different reasons. So let's go through them.

1st, 2nd and 3rd Gen

Generation one, two and three are rarely used.

1st Gen - Generation one was introduced by Dr. Michael Buonocore in 1956, when he invented the bonding agent. It was mainly for etching enamel and left the dentin and smear layer as they were.

2nd Gen - Similar to generation one, slightly better adhesive properties but still completely failed to remove the smear layer.

3rd Gen - In generation three they realised the need to remove the smear layer. However, they used unfilled resin which was very runny and ineffective at bonding composite. So they weren't very successful and they gave a bad reputation to composite material until the fourth generation bonding agent came along.

4th Gen (gold standard)

With fourth generation bonding agents there is a complete removal of the smear layer by using total etch technique, 15 to 20 seconds on dentine. The primer keeps the dentine moist to avoid collagen collapse, as we know that if you over dry dentine the collagen collapses and then you don't get the resin tags and you don't get a hybrid layer which is strong enough for you to give a high quality bond.

Generation four dentine bonding agents introduced moist bonding ensuring that the dentine doesn't dry up.

This system is very effective when used correctly and still the gold standard. Optibond FL was invented in 1995 and it's still a gold standard even though we now have eight generations of bonding agents available. This bonding agent has the best long-term clinical track record and is most versatile of all eight categories.

Hence, I advise using this bonding agent for every single direct or indirect restoration.

Here is a list of dentine bonding agents available which are fourth generation bonding agents.

Table 7:

Generation	Brand name	Manufacturer	Polymerisation
4th generation Three-steps Etch-Rinse	All-Bond 3	Bisco Schaumburg, IL, USA	Light cured, Dual
	Clearfil Liner Bond	Kuraray (Kurashiki, Japan)	Light or self-cured
	Scotchbond Multi-Purpose	(3M, ESPE, St. Paul, Minn, USA)	Light cured
	Adper Scotchbond Multi-Purpose Plus	(3M, ESPE, St. Paul, Minn, USA)	Light cured, Dual
	Optibond FL	(Kerr, Orrange, CA, USA)	Light Cured
	Gluma Solid Bond	(Heraeus Kulzer, Wehrheim, Germany)	Light Cured
	Solobond Plus	DMG, Hamburg, Germany	Light Cured
	Luxa Bond Total Etch	VOCO, Cuxhaven, Germany, DMG America	Light Cured, Dual

I advise you to have a look at them carefully because they are considered to be a gold standard; however, not all of them are the same. There are some unique differences between them, such as filler content in each adhesive.

5th Gen

Fifth generation bonding agents were invented in the 1990's, the same era as 4th generation. They were created to simplify the process. By simplifying what they did is create a single bottle system where you use etch and then use a single bottle which combines primer and bond together.

The problem here is that when you combine two acidic components together, they are not as effective and scientists realised that they were susceptible to water degradation because of the way they are fabricated and chemically composed. As a result they don't give as good results as fourth generation bonds.

These are the bonds available as a fifth generation bond.

Table 8:

Generation	Brand name	Manufacturer	Polymerisation
5th Generation Two-Steps Etch-Rinse	Solobond M	Voco (Cuxhaven, Germany)	Light cured
	Gluma One Bond	Heraeus Kulzer, Hanau, Germany	Light cured
	Optibond Solo Plus	Kerr (Orange, Calif. USA)	Light cured
	Optibond SoloPlus Dual Care	Kerr (Orange, Calif. USA)	Dual dured
	Prime&Bond 2.1	Dentsply-Detrey (Konstanz), Germany	Light cured
	Adper Single Bond Plus, (Adper Single Bond 2)	3M ESPE, St. Paul, MN, USA	Light cured
	Scotchbond 1 (Single Bond)	Kuraray (Osaka, Japan)	Light cured
	Clearfil Liner Bond 2	Kuraray (Osaka, Japan)	Light cured
	Clearfil SE	Kuraray Medical Inc (Tokyo, Japan)	Dual cured

6th Gen

The sixth generation bonding agents were invented in the late 90s and early 2000s. The innovation was self-etching primers. People thought that with total etch the teeth started getting sensitive because now dentists were etching dentine, exposing that dentine and teeth become sensitive as a result. However, in my experience teeth become sensitive because of improper techniques used for bonding.

So, the self-etching primer was invented which meant you didn't need to etch and rinse which avoided over drying and avoided causing sensitivity issues. Instead of that you mixed primer and adhesive together right before application. It is recommended that the components are mixed together just prior to application because primer has got acid in it with the etch and both mixed together at the same time just before application to keep it fresh.

The proposed advantage was that there is less dependence on the hydration stage of dentine which is true.

The disadvantage was that the pH wasn't high enough to etch enamel. As a result they started recommending that you etch and dry the enamel and then use a generation 6 bonding agent on the enamel and dentine to improve the bonding. However, it can be difficult to isolate the enamel by itself. So, dentists were etching again, defeating the whole idea behind sixth generation bonding agents.

These are different type of sixth generation bonding agents available on the market provided by different companies:

Table 9:

Generation	Brand name	Manufacturer	Polymerisation
6th Generation Two-Steps Etch-Rinse	ART Bond	Coltene (Alstatten, Switzerland)	Light cured
	Clearfil SE	Kuraray (Tokyo Japan)	Light cured
	Clearfil Protect Bond	Kuraray (Tokyo Japan)	Light cured
	Adper Scotchbond SE self-etch	3M ESPE (St. Paul, MN, USA)	Light cured
	FL bond II	Shofu Dental	Light cured
	Clearfill Liner bond 2V	Kuraray (Tokyo Japan)	Light cured
	Clearfil S3 Bond	Kuraray (Tokyo Japan)	Light cured
	G Bond	GC Corp (Tokyo, Japan)	Light cured
	iBond Gluma inside	Heraeus Kulzer (Hanau, Germany)	Light cured
	Prompt Adper Prompt L-Pop	3M ESPE (St. Paul, MN, USA)	Light cured
	L-Pop	3M ESPE (St. Paul, MN, USA)	Light cured

7th Gen

Seventh generation bonding agent is really a single-bottle self-etch primer plus bond agent. So you have a single-bottle and everything is included in there.

These inherently acidic systems tend to have a significant amount of water in their formulation so are often prone to hydrolysis and chemical breakdown.

Furthermore, once placed and polymerised they are generally more hydrophilic than two-step self-etching systems and this property makes them more prone to water absorption. This has the same limitations as the other bond where you mix prime and bond together and it limits the depth of resin infiltration into the tooth.

8th Gen

8th generation bonding agents are very similar to the 7th generation. However, they contain nano sized particles and create a thicker hybrid layer, arguably because of the nano-sized particles; however, there is not much research out there because it's relatively new.

These are the seventh and eighth generation bonding agents.

Table 10:

Generation	Brand name	Manufacturer	Polymerisation
7/8th Generation One-step Self-Etch	One Coat 7.0	Coltène/Whaledent (AG, Altstätten, Switzerland)	Light cured
	AdheSE One F (no mix)	Ivoclar Vivadent, (Schaan, Principality of Liechtenstein)	Light cured
	G-BOND	GC America (Alsip, IL, USA)	Light cured
	OptiBond All-In-One	Kerr (Orange, CA, USA)	Light cured
	Clearfil S3 Bond Plus	Kuraray (Tokyo, Japan)	Light cured
	Adper Easy one	3M ESPE (St. Paul, Minn. USA)	Light cured
	Clearfill DC bond	Kuraray (Tokyo, Japan)	Dual cured

Then you have universal bonding agents which are used for every purpose and you can use whichever way you want to use them.

These are the bonding agents which are universal bonding agents.

Table 11:

Generation	Brand name	Manufacturer	Polymerisation
Multimode or Universal	Prime&Bond Elect	Dentsply Caulk (Milford, DE, USA)	Light cured
	AdheSe Universal	Ivoclar Vivadent (Schaan, Principality of Liechtenstein)	Light cured
	G-aenial bond	GC America (Alsip, IL, USA)	Light cured
	Clearfil Universal Bond	Kuraray (Tokyo, Japan)	Light cured, self cured
	Scotchbond Universal	3M ESPE (St. Paul, Minn. USA)	Light cured

As you can see there are lots of bonding agents available on the market. It can be confusing working out which one to use because if you go to any brand of fourth to eighth generation bonding agent, they will all naturally say that their bonding agent is the best.

So how would you determine which bonding agent is best? We will come to that in a minute.

Classification by mechanism of adhesion

- a **three-step technique** where you etch prime and bond. This is still a gold standard.
- a **two-step technique** (version 1).
  In step one of which you etch the tooth and then in step two you have a bottle with the prime and bond together.
- a **two-step technique** (version 2).
  Step one is when you apply self-etching primer and then the bond, which comes in a separate bottle, as a step two.
- There is another technique where it's a **one step** where everything's included in one bottle.

Practical properties

What are practical (which can be used in a day to day practice) properties one should look out for in a bonding agent?

- **Radiopaque**
  Practically we want our bond to be radiopaque because we want to be able to distinguish between our bonds and caries. If I've removed the caries before bonding something I need to make sure that I haven't left any caries behind. If my bond is radiolucent then on an x-ray there is always confusion whether the junction showing between composite and a tooth is a bond or a caries or whether my comp is not adapting properly to the floor of the cavity. So I want my bond to be radiopaque.

- **Removal of smear layer**
  I would prefer to remove the smear layer completely to enhance my bonding. But at the same time I do not want sensitivity to be an issue.

- **Highly filled**
  I want it to be highly filled because I want to be able to apply a thick layer of the bond. Again, when we discuss IDS (Immediate Dentine Sealing) it will become clearer why when choosing a bond I am considering these three categories.

Best bonding agent

So, what is the best bond in my opinion? Fourth generation bonds are known to be a gold standard. If everyone's saying that the fourth generation bond is a gold standard why move away from that fourth generation bond?

We have enough evidence to show that fourth generation bonds still work and until I see robust data demonstrating a batter practice then I am sticking with them.

As I said before, not all fourth generation bonds are the same and my favourite bond is OptiBond FL. I have been using this bond since 2011 and with an excellent success rate. Having said that, I know many dentists who use different bonds and they are happy with them.

So whatever bonding system you're using, make sure that you understand the principles and if it works in your hands then fair enough. Just use that bond because I don't want you to change something when what you have is already working well for you. Having said that, if you change to something new you will encounter challenges in the beginning, not because the product is difficult only because you are new to it. The most important thing is to make sure that you feel comfortable in using whatever you're using.

I would like to make it clear that I do not have a personal interest in any specific product nor do I get paid to promote any products.

IDS (Immediate Dentine Sealing)

- Immediate dentine sealing is sealing the dentine straight after it is freshly cut to avoid any contamination. We know from the studies that when you seal the dentine when it is freshly cut and if it's not contaminated you get the best hybrid layer. This means you get the best bond to that dentine when bonding final restoration and that is called Immediate Dentine Sealing.
- This is usually used for indirect restoration because with direct restoration you're preparing the cavity and you're sealing the dentine and you're doing your restoration on top at the same time.
- For indirect restoration, where you are preparing the tooth, temporising it, leaving it for a few weeks, days or even hours and then cementing or bonding your indirect restoration.
- So Immediate Dentine Sealing is for any indirect restoration. What we are trying to aim for is to seal that dentine as soon as you have finished cutting and removing all the debris from it.

Advantages of IDS

- One of the main advantages is **patient comfort** during provisionalisation. I used to have so many sensitivity complaints during provisionalisation and I used to have to tell them to wait until we had bonded the final restoration. Since I started doing IDS, I no longer have this issue. Sometimes patients complain a little bit about sensitivity, however, this only happens when my IDS wasn't done properly. Even when patients have complained, the sensitivity is nowhere nearly as severe as before.
- You have **less need for anaesthesia**. Fit appointments are much more convenient for the patient. 60% of my onlay fits are done without any local anaesthetic. Sometimes I give local anaesthetic because patients don't like clamps when placing a rubber dam so I give a local anaesthetic just to numb the gum. Generally patients don't have tooth sensitivity even after I've removed the temporary. They rarely feel any sensitivity even when I am sandblasting the tooth and cleaning.
- It **reduces post bonding or cementation sensitivity** and **increases the bond strength.** As discussed above we are sealing the dentine there and then, so we are creating the hybrid layer while the dentine is fresh and not contaminated. This gives the best result when you bond the restoration a few weeks later.

- Treating dentine and enamel independently gives you the best result because you're rebuilding the substructure in the way it is naturally available.

Procedure: Preparation appointment (if tooth needs composite build up)

Let's look at best practice protocol for immediate dentine sealing during the whole procedure from the preparation to the fit.

Procedure: Preparation appointment

- If you are preparing a tooth on the preparation appointment, you prepare the tooth as you normally do.
- You then need to identify the dentine and you can do this by etching the whole tooth for two seconds and drying it, so then you know where the enamel is so you can leave that alone.
- Then etch dentine for around 15 seconds. Wash etch for 20 seconds.
- Apply the primer for 20 seconds and rub the primer really nicely to make sure it's penetrating. Sometimes you need to apply primer twice. Do this once you are sure that you have wetted the surface really well.
- Dry the primer out very gently leaving a moist surface. Drying or using suction on the primer is very important because you want to remove the acetone which is there on the primer. You need to remove that before you put the adhesive bond on it because if you left that acetone and you haven't dried, the bond won't work very well. However, if you over dry it then the primer may not function. It is a critical skill to be able to dry just enough to leave the area shiny and moist but not so moist that you still have the acetone in it.
- Finally, you apply adhesive to your dentine.

When you're doing that, you need to make sure your bond is more than 42 microns thick because the oxygen inhibition layer is 42 microns. Now if you imagine your bond is 10, 11 microns thick, it has got that inhibition layer and hence it never cures, and ultimately IDS fails. If you do not have a filled bond and if the only option you have is to use an unfilled bond, you need to protect this bond using composite on top of this bond.

However, it is not an issue with OptiBond FL. You can get a thick layer of the OptiBond FL. If the area is small then you can use a tip of the probe to apply a bond. However, make sure the probe doesn't touch the dentine otherwise you can damage the nicely prepared surface and just drop the bond in the area with the probe.

Sometimes you cannot avoid bonding to enamel. That's okay because at the end of the process we're going to freshen the enamel anyway, so I wouldn't worry too much about the bond going on to the enamel though try and avoid this if you can.

- Then you light the cure.
- Then you are going to place glycerin on top and then cure it again.
- Then you use pumice and polishing brushes to clean the area to remove even smaller layers of that oxygen inhibition layer.
- Once that's done you refresh the enamel with the round bur or something fine. However, avoid going into the dentine and make sure your bur stays onto the dentine.
- Then you take the impression and temporise the tooth.

If you are using some sort of a temporary composite material you must use Vaseline on your preparation before you use that temporary composite material. Otherwise that will stick to the tooth even though you've used glycerin and pumice, there is still a good chance that your temporary material might stick to your bond which is applied to the dentine. We know that eugenol based temporary cements inhibit the final bonding and hence it is best to avoid those temporary cements.

So just make sure that you apply a little bit of vaseline as a separating medium and then use your temporary composite material.

Above protocol is a pure IDS protocol where we are not using any composite. Immediate Dentine Sealing (IDS) does not involve using composite if you use Opt Bond FL, unless you have an unfilled bond. However, many times we need to block undercut or do DME (deep marginal elevation) after the preparation. This involves using composite after using a bonding agent. In this case, you will use bond and composite wherever it is needed, including enamel, and make sure if any remaining dentine is covered with a bonding agent. Once you finish that, glycerine, air block it, pumice to clean and then freshen the enamel if any enamel is exposed, and then do an impression apply vaseline and temporise.

Procedure: Fit appointment

Now we are going to look at what happens in the fit appointment.

There are two different protocols for the fit appointment: one for bonding composite or hybrid onlays and another one for porcelain onlays or for porcelain restorations.

Treating the fitting surface of the indirect composite onlay or veneer:

- First use a micro etcher/sandblaster on the fitting surface.
- Etch for 90 seconds then rinse with phosphoric acid. Etching doesn't really do anything to the composite, the reason etching is necessary is to clean the surface properly to remove particles from sand blasters. So etch to remove all the debris.
- Next, apply silane on the fit surface and heat treat composite silane. You can use a small wax heater or a hair dryer to heat the silane. If you don't heat treat the silane, the efficacy of the adhesion will be significantly reduced.
- Once that is heat treated, apply some adhesive bond on to the fitting surface just before fitting. Do not cure the bond.
- Last, we will apply heated composite onto the onlay which we have prepared and take it to the tooth for fitting.

Treating the fitting surface of the porcelain crown/onlay/veneer:

- If you are using porcelain, avoid sand blasting. Instead, etch using 9-10% hydrofluoric acid for 90 seconds when working with feldspathic porcelain. Use 4-5% hydrofluoric acid for 20 seconds when working with lithium disilicate.
- Next we are going to wash it and put it in a sonic alcohol bath.
- Then we apply porcelain silane and heat treat it.
- We coat it with adhesive resin just before we apply it onto the tooth. Do not cure the adhesive resin.
- Lastly we will put the heated composite onto the fitting surface of the restoration before fitting it onto the tooth.

You can see that I am suggesting using heated composite for all bonding protocols. What I have described is a heated restorative composite. If you are not comfortable using this method then you can use panavia, a similar dual cure or highly filled resin material. However, heated composite is best practice in my professional opinion especially for veneers (unless they are very thin) and onlays. It can be difficult to use for crowns and hence you can stick with conventional methods of bonding or cementing. I would urge all of you to try this technique.

Not all composites heat as well as we would like, so you need to be able to figure out whether the composite you're using is good for this technique by trying it out on a model first.

Treating the fitting surface of the tooth:

With regards to preparing the tooth, we will be refreshing the adhesive by using a diamond burr or a micro etcher/sandblaster. Most of the time I use a micro etcher because I find it to be much more precise. Then we use total etch on enamel, dentine and composite whichever we are dealing with for 30 seconds. Because we haven't exposed dentine there is no need to worry. However, sometimes when you're using a micro etcher you might expose dentine.

So what to do if you have exposed dentine?

I would etch dentine for 15 seconds and the rest of it for 30 seconds. Then we use a primer for 20 seconds and gently rub around the area.

Then apply an adhesive bonding agent. I would not cure the bond on the tooth.

Then I would use heated composite as above on the restoration, place the restoration on the tooth, make sure you apply a lot of pressure then remove all excess then apply pressure again and remove excess, repeat this several times and then cure the whole block in one go, once you are sure that restoration has seated well.

Heated composites allow us to remove all the excess material before curing the composites so it gives us plenty of time so we can do our best work. There is no time constraint unlike if you're using dual cure material or even light cure. Flowable composite can be difficult to use because it's quite runny. If you use dual cure then as we discussed above, it starts setting quickly, so you are working under time pressure. Hence, a restorative composite is better for many reasons. The lack of time pressure both enables you to do better work and makes your job less stressful.

Tools:

Let's look at some of the tools I use for my direct adhesive reconstruction which I would advise you to use or at least have it in mind so that when you need to buy again you may want to just try these tools out.

Disclaimer: I am not affiliated with any company.

- **Rubber Dam - Non latex, medium dam**
  I normally use a medium non-latex rubber dam as it makes my work both much easier and of a higher standard. Less tear, makes it much easier to isolate and looks nice on the photographs.

- **Rubber Dam clamps + Holder + Punch**
  You need clamps. Here is a wide selection of clamps and we need to use hygiene products for them. And they have plenty of clamps. There are some clamps which are wingless which you may have to buy separately or sometimes you may need to section

the anterior clamp in order to get two sort of separate clamps but that's something you will not be able to buy anywhere you need to fabricate your own version of the clamps.

- **Rubberdam METAL frame**
  The other kit comes with a plastic frame. I don't like plastic frames, so I have metal frames (***Figure 88***) which are far sturdier and they hold the rubber much more precisely.

FIGURE 88

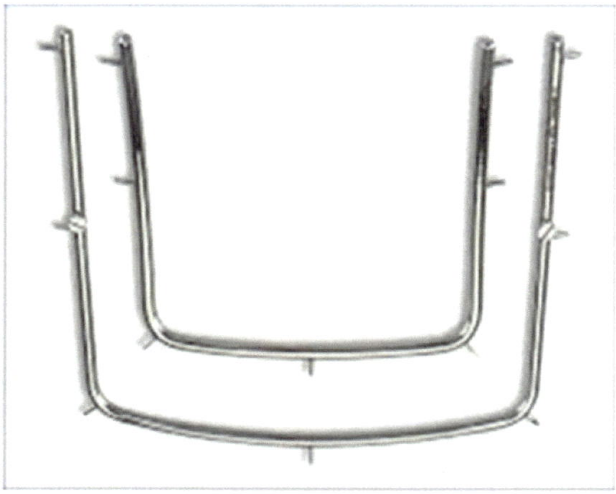

- **OptiBond FL**
  As I have said, my favoured bonding agent is OptiBond FL. (***Figure 89***). It enables my bonding technique to be much more effective and improves my success rate.

FIGURE 89

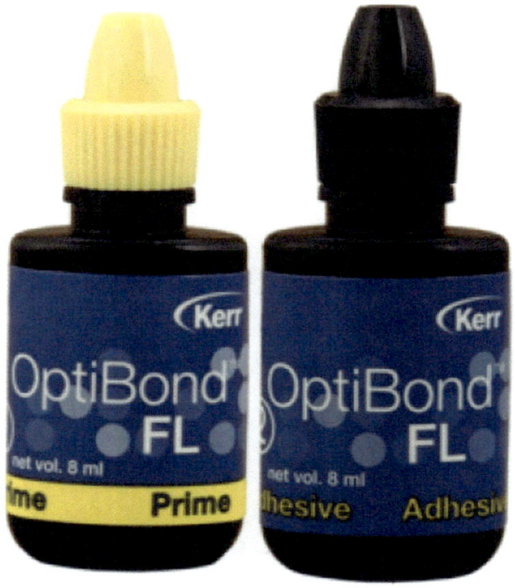

- **PTFE tape**
  I use PTFE (***Figure 90***) to isolate teeth by covering either side of the teeth. If I'm bonding one tooth in order to make sure that my composite doesn't get stuck to the other teeth, and also so that my etch and everything associated with it doesn't affect the enamel and dentine of the other teeth. PTFE tape is something you will be using often.

FIGURE 90

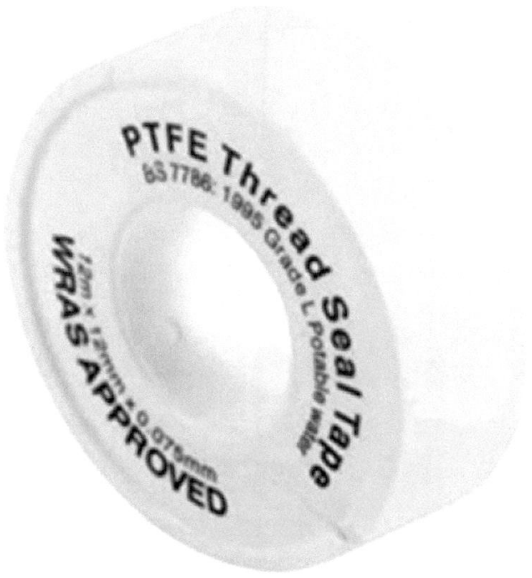

- **Composite**
  Regarding composite, there are many brands to choose from. I mostly use composite dentine and enamel shade. If I'm using any staining then it's mainly white staining.

- **Clear inter proximal strips**
  Clear, see-through, mylar strips are very useful. They enable me to see what's going on while I am adapting the treatment I am doing.

- **Instruments**
  I have done full mouth adhesive technique by just using a probe and amalgam carver. However, if you want fancy instruments then here are the instruments I use. I use LM art instruments. These are really nice, ergonomic and have very fine tips.

  One of the instrument in the kit has got a blade like cutting edge so you can remove some of the excess material very easily. This is useful because sometimes the number 12 blade is very difficult to get to in some areas.

- **Glycerin Jelly (thick in consistency)**
  Glycerine air blocker. We know from the text above that glycerin, as an air blocker is a must for any bonding procedure.

- **Interproximal Serrated Strips**
  This is another must. Interproximal serrated strips are metal strips **(*Figure 91*)**. These strips will help you a lot. Let us say you are building up six anterior teeth, you will inevitably bond two teeth to each other, it may be very slight but you will end up bonding them. You can use this strip to separate them easily.

FIGURE 91

If you were to use regular interproximal strips with posterior teeth there is a chance that you will cut the patient's lip. There are specialised strips with safety handles to use with posterior teeth (***Figure 92***). These make your work easier for you and safer for your patient.

FIGURE 92

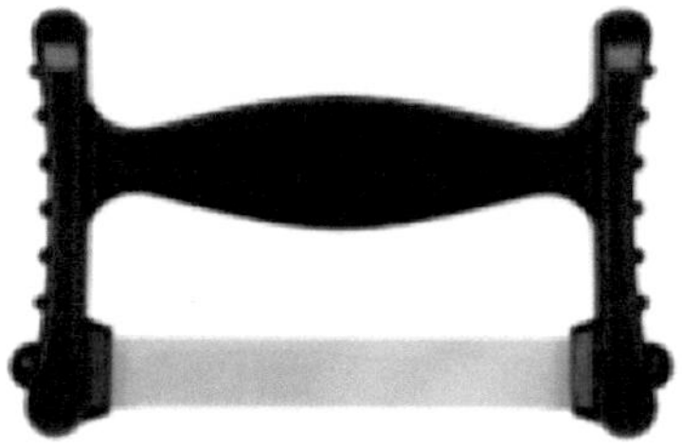

- **No 12 and No 11 blades**
  Number 12 blades are perfect to remove the excess material from the interproximal area once you build up the teeth. Number 11 is to cut your indices and make sure everything is nice and tidy. These two blades are my go-to blades.

FIGURE 93

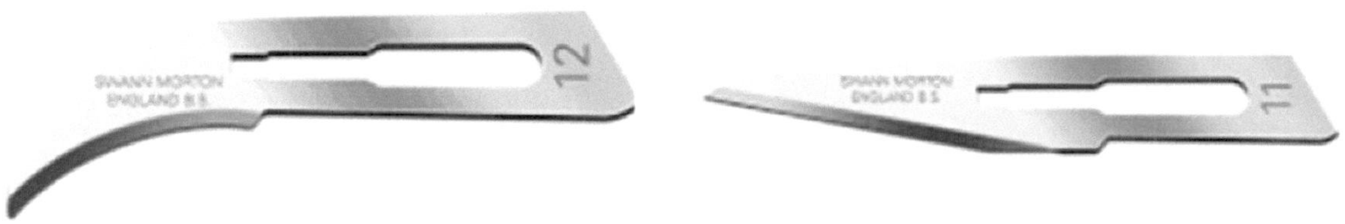

- **Composite polishing strips**
  I use metal composite polishing strips and only use a yellow strip because otherwise if you use them quite harshly you can open up the contact. I don't tend to use it near the contact area. I would go right near the gum area and I will just clean the embrasures really nicely so they help the patient in using interdental brushes and keeping it clean.

- **Selection of burs for polishing**
  There is a wide selection of burs to choose from. You probably have your own burs already.

- **Composite polishing discs**
  These are the polishing discs we have at the practice and they work really well. With polishing discs I use the coarse ones first and then the medium ones. That's all, the remaining polishing is done via polishing burs and wheels.

- **Composite polishing wheels**
  I would use an A.S.A.P. bur to polish my composite really well. If these are not available then you can use venus supra kit.

  Hopefully this has helped you understand the tools available which will enable you to do high quality full mouth reconstructions easily and reliably.

3.2 Anterior Direct Build Up

Treatment flow for adhesive DIRECT full mouth reconstruction

Before we go ahead and discuss anterior direct buildup, let's recap the steps involved in direct reconstruction.

As we discussed above, step one is treatment planning. Step two is anterior reconstruction. Step three is posterior reconstruction.

Step 1: Treatment planning

In the section on treatment planning we discussed comprehensive assessment, impression and record taking, mounting in CR, CO, or ICP, diagnostic wax up and using mockups for the patient to try out and confirm the plan.

Step 2: Anterior build ups

In anterior buildups we are building upper and lower anterior teeth with definitive direct composite and we are then stabilising posterior teeth.

Step 3: Posterior build ups

In posterior buildup we will be doing posterior definitive restorations. We do this one arch at a time or one side at a time. We protect the teeth once we have finished the treatment and then establish the maintenance protocol.

Anterior build ups

In this section we are going to concentrate on step two. Let's look at this step more in detail.

Anterior buildup can be done in many ways; using direct, indirect, semi-direct or direct-indirect methodology.

Direct method

In the direct method, you have freehand build up, a putty index technique and a clear index technique. You can use Memosil or Exaclear. Currently all my build ups are done using Exaclear. Memosil is not clear but it was the best material for its time. Now however, Exaclear (product from GC), a product that is clear and see-through, has come on the market. This is really handy and enables a higher standard of dental care. You can also use the injection moulding technique or you can use the SmileFast technique which is used in the UK. My preferred method is using Exaclear as an index for free hand and for stamp technique.

Indirect method

The indirect method is best used when your palatal build up is going to have a thickness of two millimetres or more. You can build teeth in composite, ceramic or even gold as well. If you are doing the crown for these teeth then you can incorporate the palatal ramp into the crown.

Direct indirect method

If you want really nice porcelain on the anterior teeth for cosmetic reasons, but don't want to destroy the tooth in order to make a crown then you can use the direct-indirect method. Using this method, we place a composite on the palatal area, and then we raise the occlusal vertical dimension, get the occlusion right and finally place porcelain on the buccal. This will reduce the aggressive wear you may get if you have a porcelain crown in the upper arch facing composite on the lower arch. So this can ensure a resilient and long lasting treatment, with excellent cosmetic value. This even prevents the particularly aggressive wear you can get with an especially bruxist patient.

Clear index using Memosil or Exaclear works

Now let's look at how the clear index using Memosil or Exaclear works.

In ***Figure 94*** this patient came to me with wear on his anterior teeth.

FIGURE 94

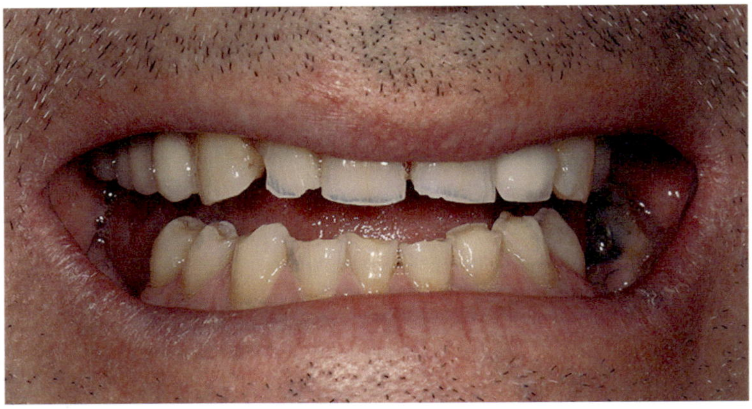

He had an upper left lateral incisor tooth implant. That was our limiting factor. As we discuss in the treatment planning chapter, you need to know if there is a limiting factor such as an implant which we have to work around. The patient didn't want to change the crown of that implant because he did not know the make of the implant.

Figure 95a shows a close smile and ***Figure 95b*** shows a retracted view.

FIGURE 95a

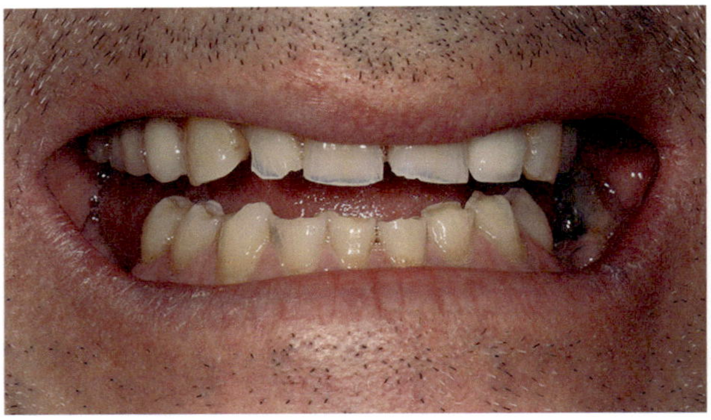

FIGURE 95b

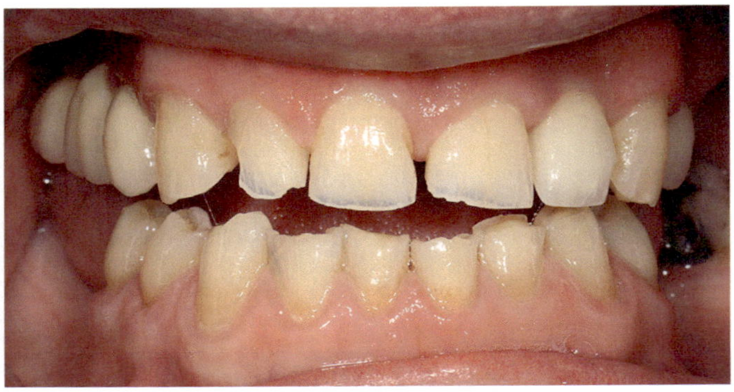

So we decided to work around the implant. This becomes a limiting factor because at the moment all his teeth are in occlusion. And if we raise OVD all the rest of the teeth can be made in occlusion but as we are not changing UL2, we may not be able to get it in occlusion.

Figure 96a shows a maxillary occlusal view and, ***Figure 96b*** shows the mandibular occlusal view.

FIGURE 96a

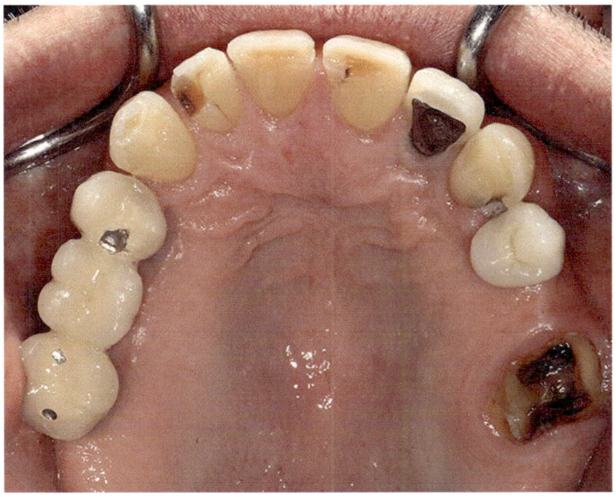

FIGURE 96b

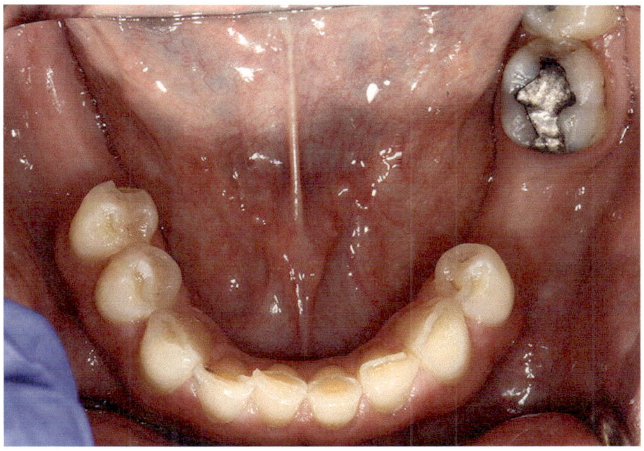

So we decided to do a wax up. After wax up I decided that we could achieve the result we wanted at increased OVD.

In ***Figure 97*** and ***Figure 98*** you can see my wax up. If I am doing a direct build up then I do all my mounting and all my wax ups so everything in these pictures was done by me.

FIGURE 97

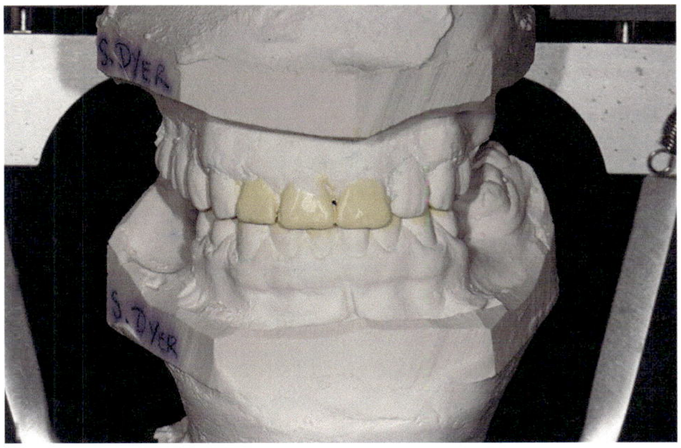

FIGURE 98

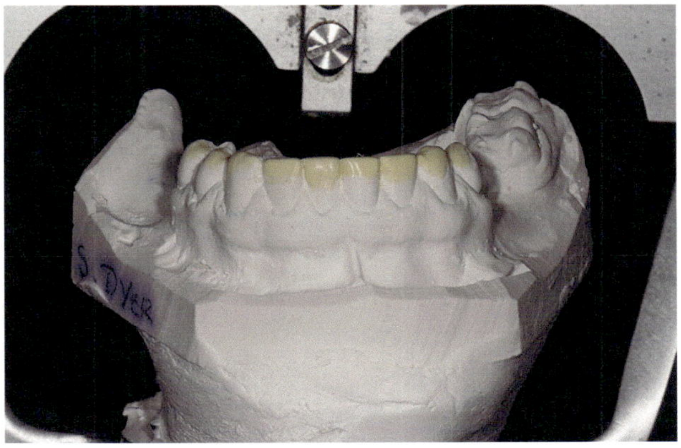

Because he had almost edge to edge occlusion, palatally we couldn't add much. There is nothing much to add on the cingulum ramp. As you can see (***Figure 99***) with the upper left implant tooth there is nothing added on that tooth because we cannot add composite to the implant. Also remember, this wax up is done only for canine to canine, once I try this in for initial approval, I then wax up the whole mouth.

FIGURE 99

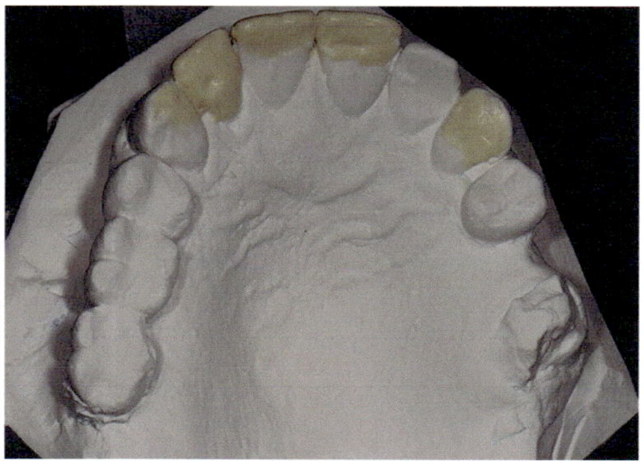

In ***Figure 100*** I isolated each tooth using floss ties.

FIGURE 100

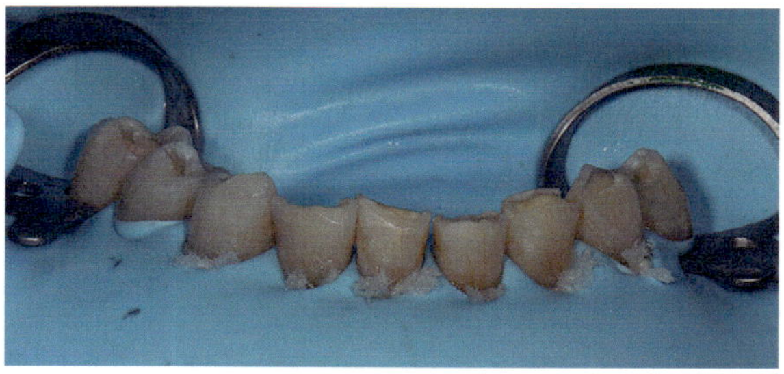

Nowadays I would do floss ties on the lingual to keep the knots away from my bonding areas. With this method it doesn't get in my way in the buccal area. Although, having said that you can see from the wax up that the wax wasn't extending all the way to the cervical area. So I wasn't too worried about that.

Figure 101 shows an occlusal view of isolation using floss ties. At this point, in ***Figure 102***, I am using Mamosil.

FIGURE 101

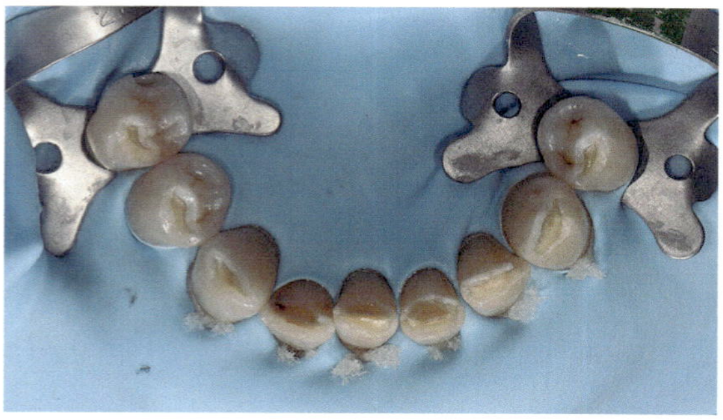

FIGURE 102

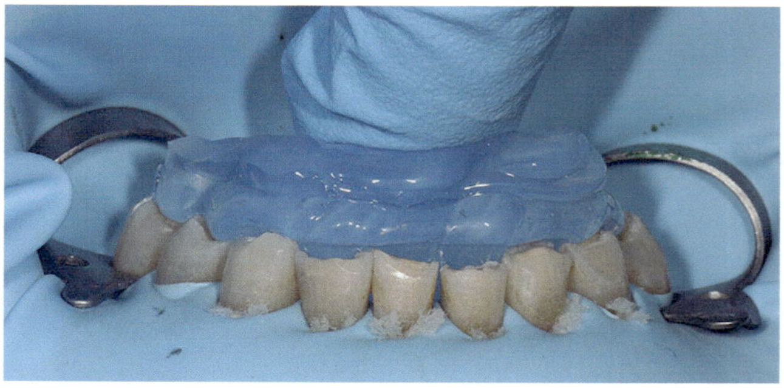

I would isolate the alternative teeth at a time as shown in ***Figure 103a*** and ***Figure 103b.***

FIGURE 103a

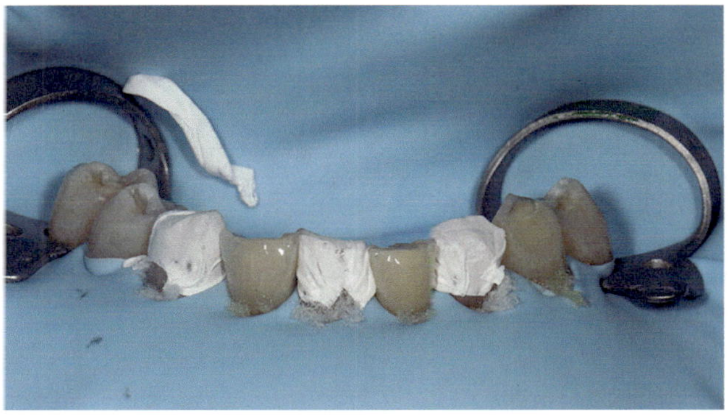

FIGURE 103b

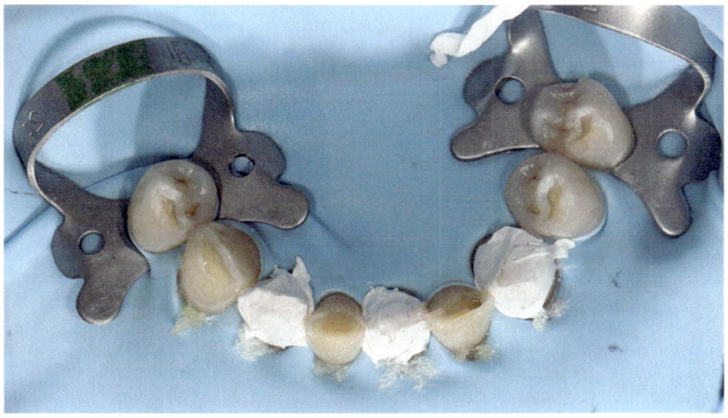

You could build the shelf of all the teeth together rather than doing alternate teeth like shown in ***Figure 104***. However, if you aren't careful then they tend to get stuck to each other.

FIGURE 104

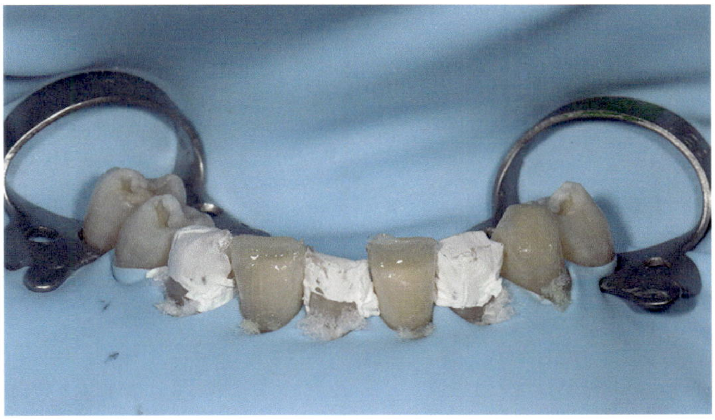

If you are adjusting the composite mid-treatment, if teeth have stuck together, that creates debris and then this debris can get into your bond. The bond then will be less effective and secure than they could be.

So I prefer to use alternative teeth. However, if you want to speed up the process and you are comfortable being very meticulous, then there is no reason why you cannot do all the teeth together.

Figure 105 shows the finished build up of the first three teeth before polishing. **Figure 106** shows PTFE on the other three teeth after building of the first three teeth.

FIGURE 105

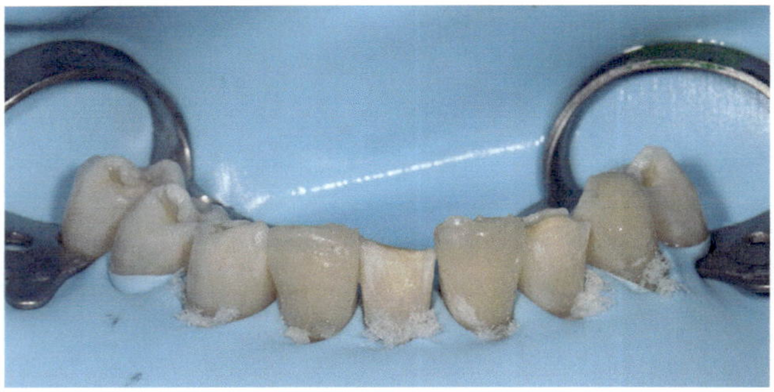

FIGURE 106

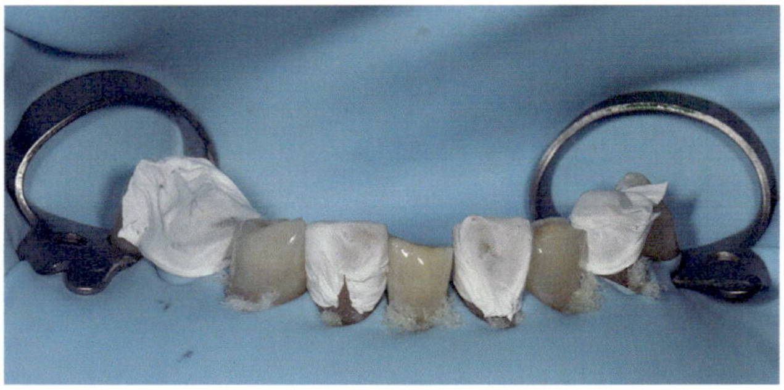

Figure 107 shows lingual shelf built up for the remaining 3 teeth.

FIGURE 107

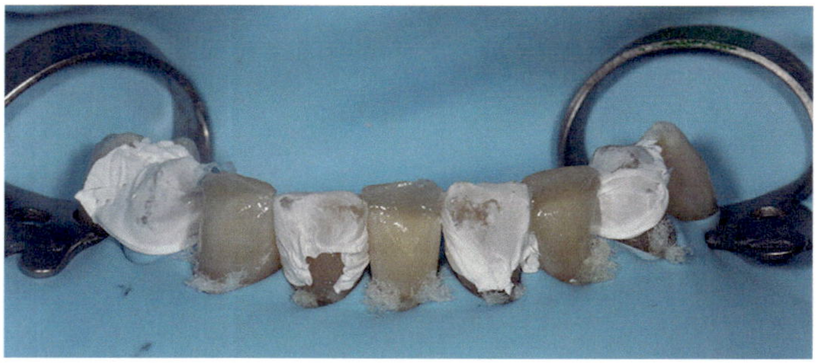

And then just do a rough polishing of the teeth.

Figure 108a shows the finished composite before polishing, and ***Figure 108b*** shows the finished composite before polishing in occlusal view.

FIGURE 108a

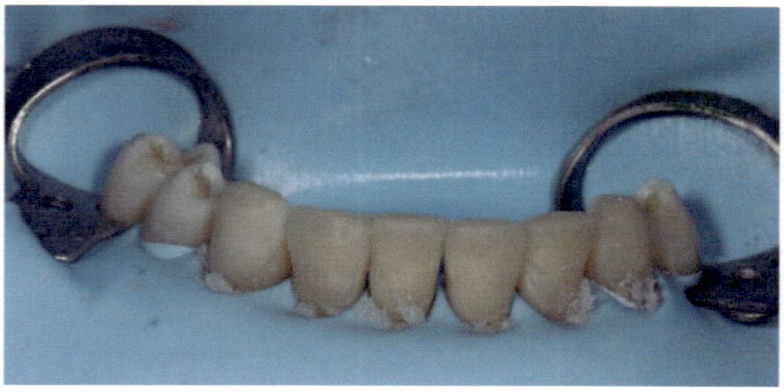

FIGURE 108b

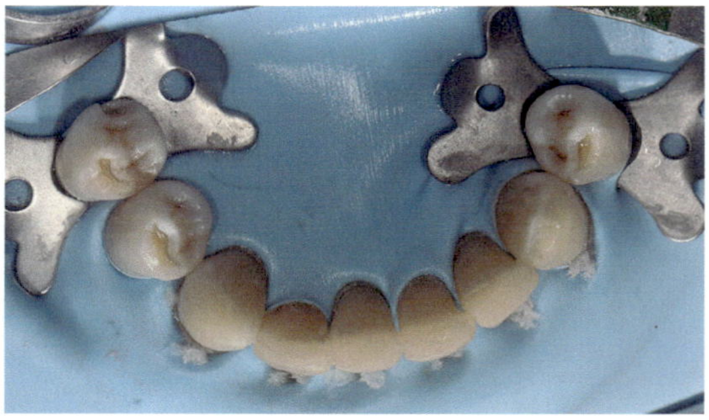

Next comes checking the occlusion as seen in ***Figure 109***.

FIGURE 109

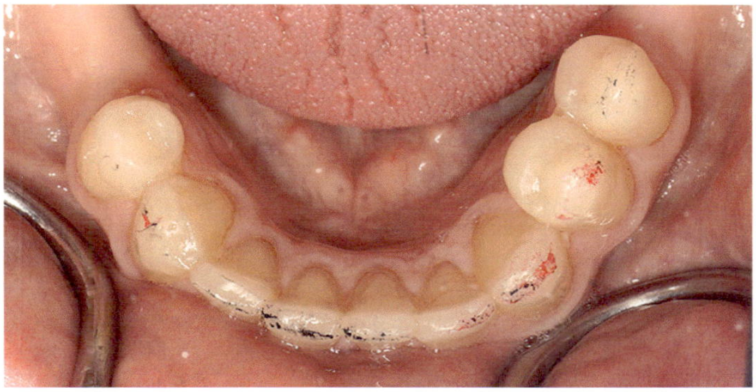

Next comes going on the opposing arch, and isolating the upper teeth, photograph taken the same day (***Figure 110***). ***Figure 111*** shows the final photo after build up.

FIGURE 110

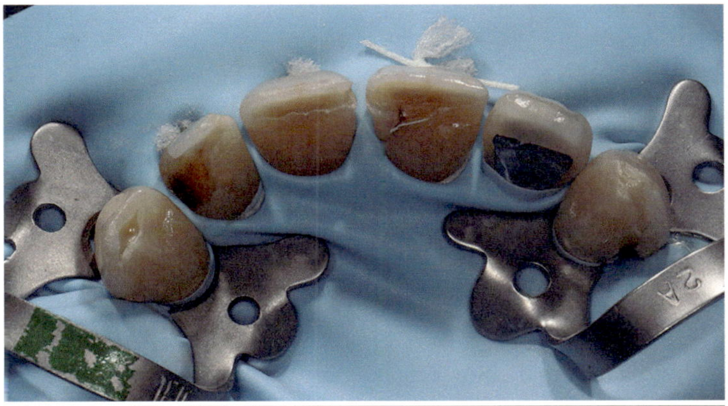

FIGURE 111

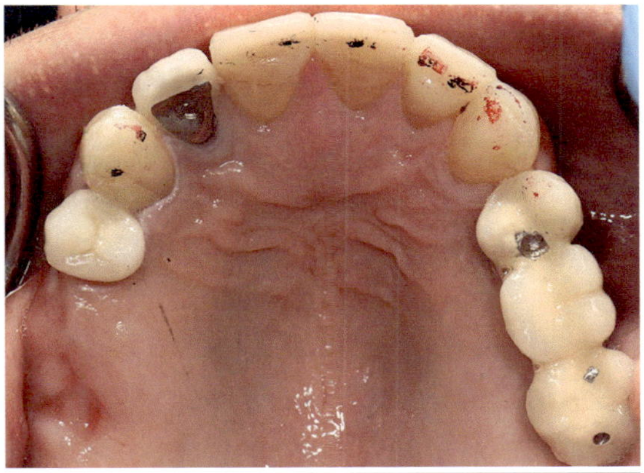

Then polishing and refining the composite.

FIGURE 112

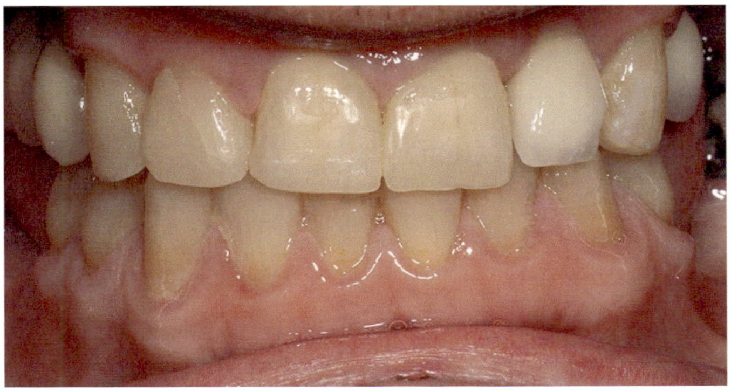

Figure 112 shows you a very straightforward anterior reconstruction. At the same time I did direct build up of the premolars as well to keep them in occlusion. ***Figure 113a*** shows the patient before the reconstruction, and ***Figure 113b*** shows the patient after the reconstruction.

FIGURE 113a

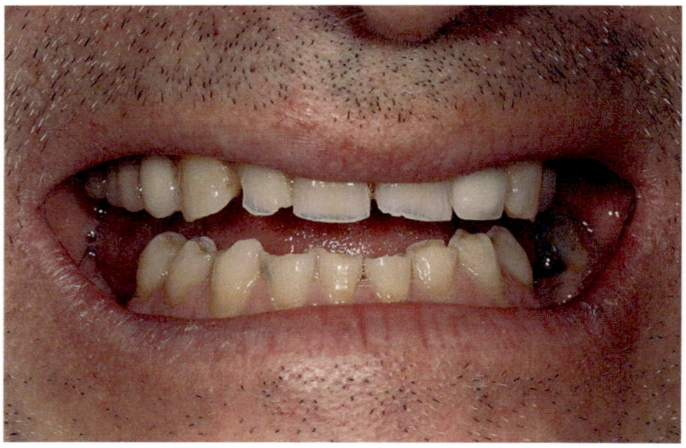

FIGURE 113b

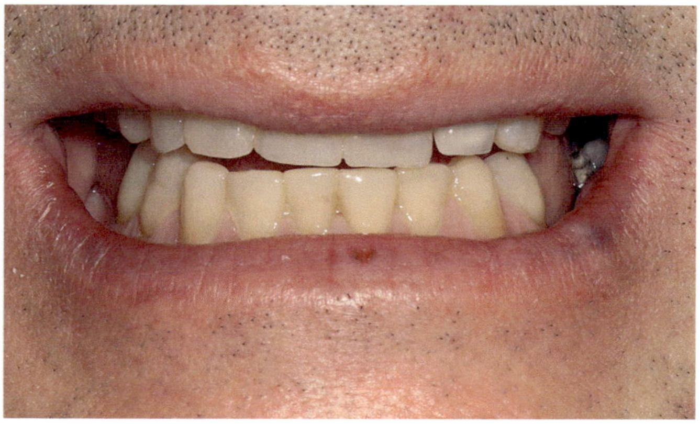

I hope these photographs help you understand how the process fits together.

Anterior build up using clear stent

Here in ***Figure 114*** is a similar lower anterior case. It is the same case as shown in ***Figure 56a*** and ***Figure 56b.***

This time I use exaclear. ***Figure 115*** shows checking the fit of Exaclear, Again I do three teeth at a time. ***Figure 116a*** shows alternative teeth isolation, ***Figure 116b*** shows building shelf for alternative teeth, ***Figure 116c*** shows the rough finishing of three teeth after build up, ***Figure 116d*** illustrates moving on to next 2 teeth as LL3 is a crown and checking index for fit, ***Figure 116e*** shows isolating 3 teeth with PTFE.

FIGURE 114

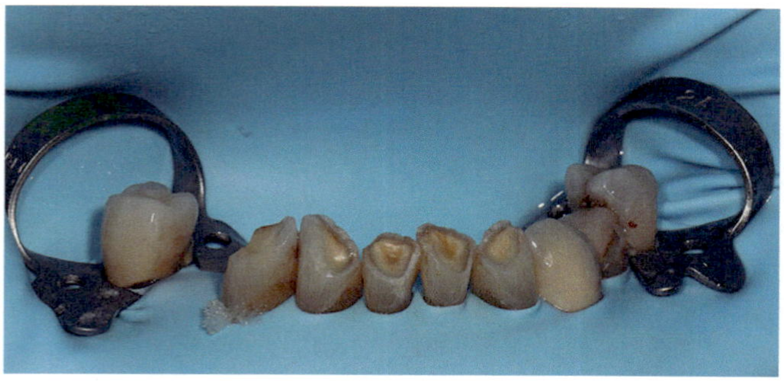

FIGURE 115

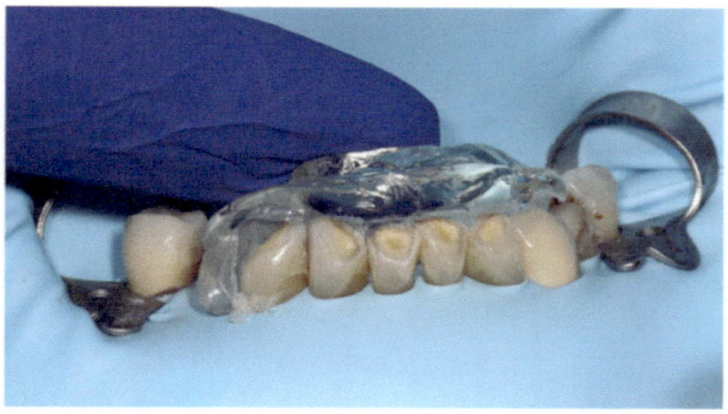

FIGURE 116a

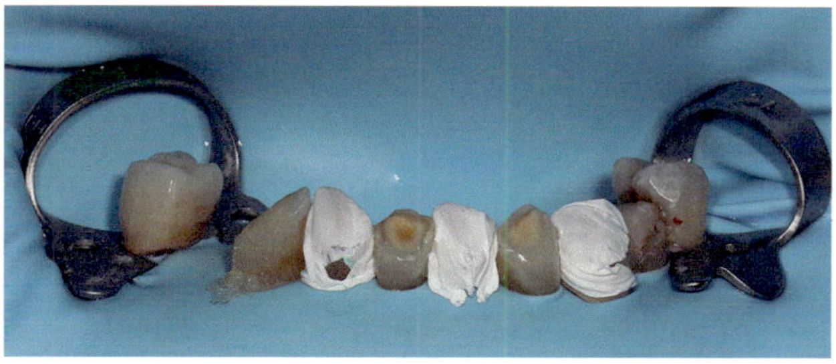

FIGURE 116b

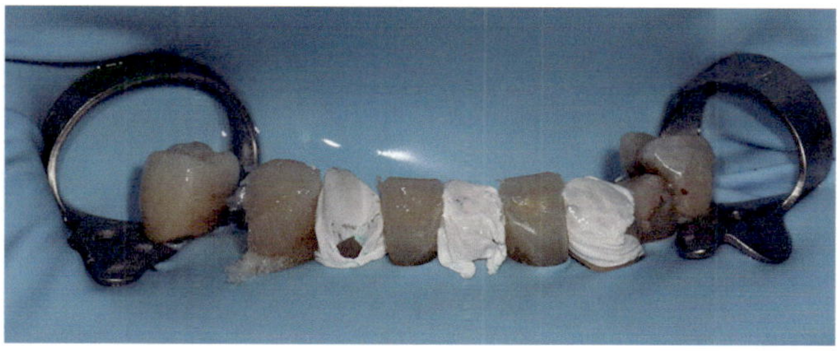

FIGURE 116c

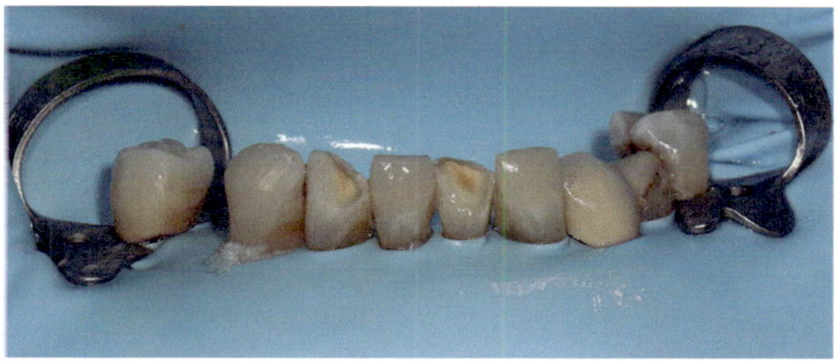

FIGURE 116d

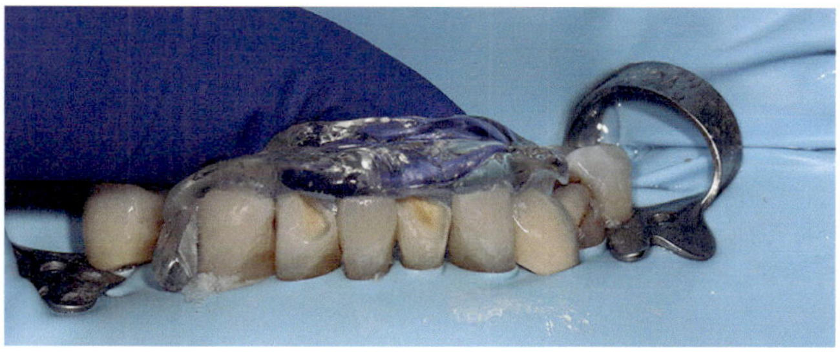

FIGURE 116e

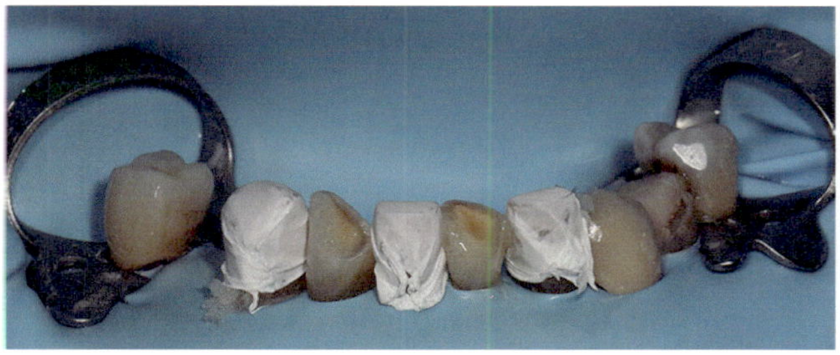

FIGURE 117

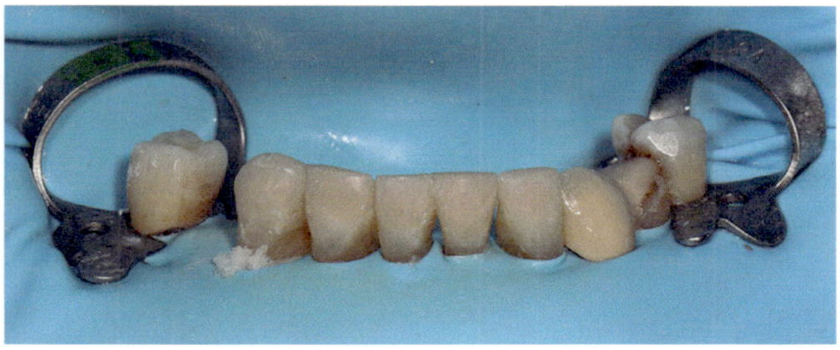

Next I do a rough polishing. ***Figure 117*** is a finished build up.
Next comes fine polishing (***Figure 118***) and finished build up.

FIGURE 118

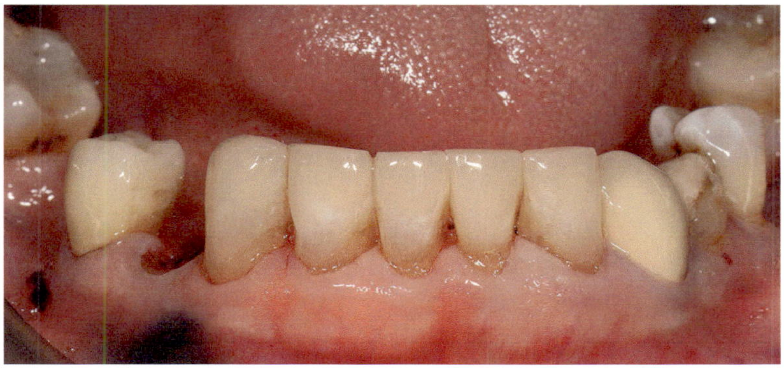

Here are the maxillary teeth of the same patient. ***Figure 119*** shows the isolation, and in ***Figure 120*** I finished the treatment. In ***Figure 120a*** shows finished maxillary build up**.**

FIGURE 119

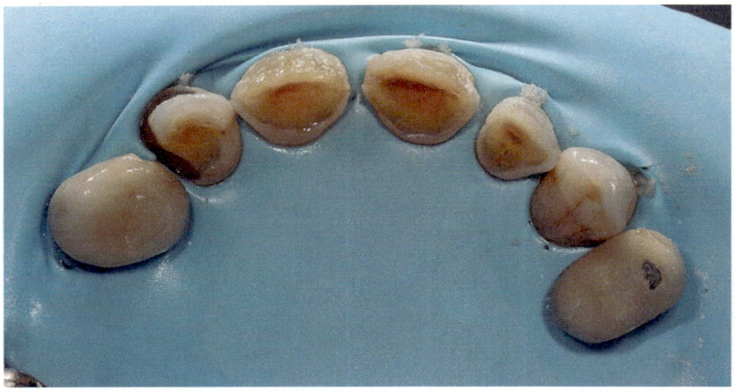

FIGURE 120a

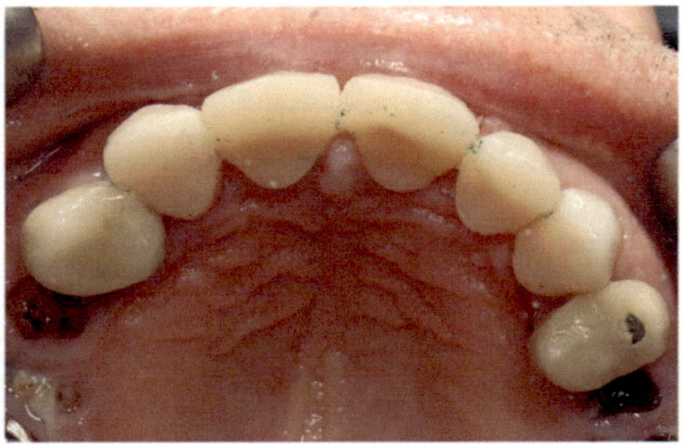

Figure 120b shows the patient before the reconstruction and ***Figure 120c*** shows the patient after reconstruction. ***Figure 120d*** shows the replacement of posterior teeth with dentures.

FIGURE 120b

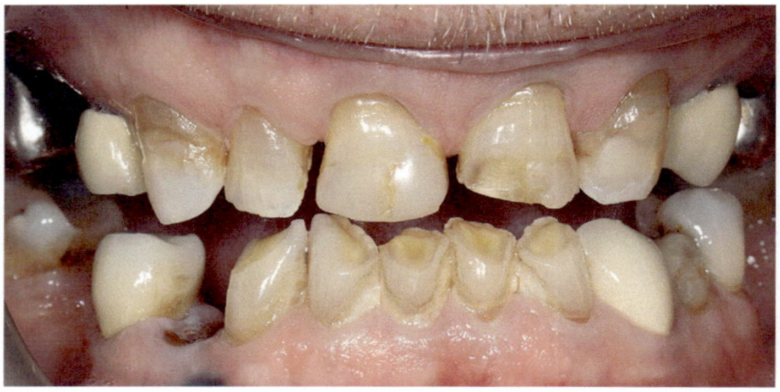

FIGURE 120c

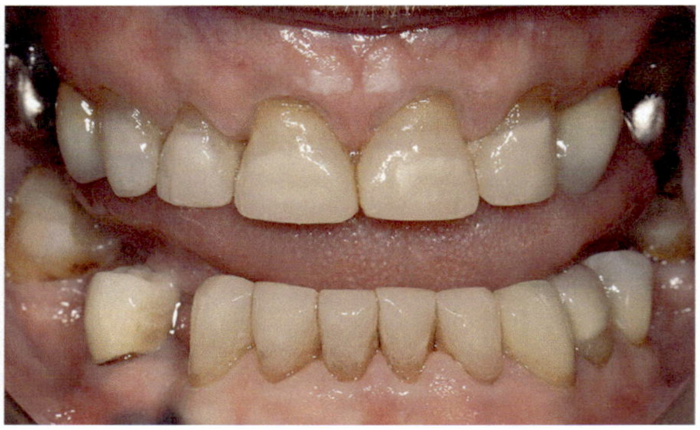

FIGURE 120d

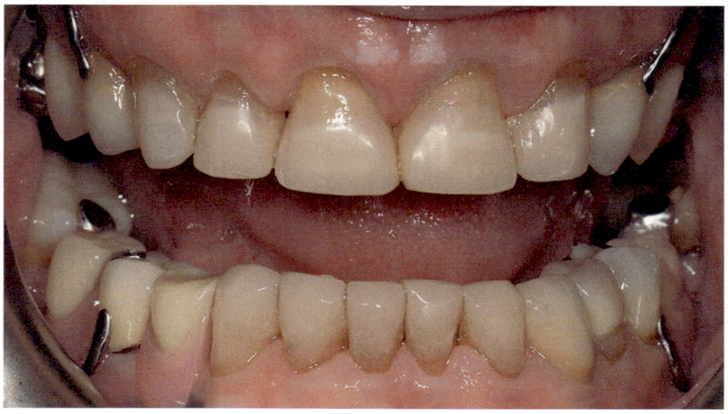

Below you can see another patient with a similar situation. ***Figure 121a*** shows the pre-op photos, ***Figure 121b*** shows the isolation, ***Figure 122*** shows the finished build up of lower anterior teeth.

FIGURE 121a

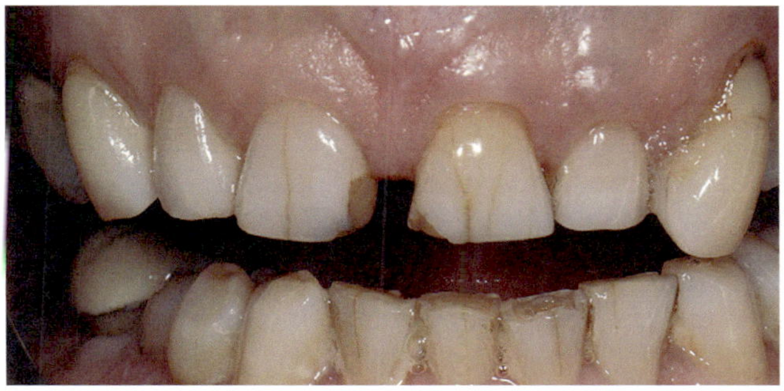

FIGURE 121b

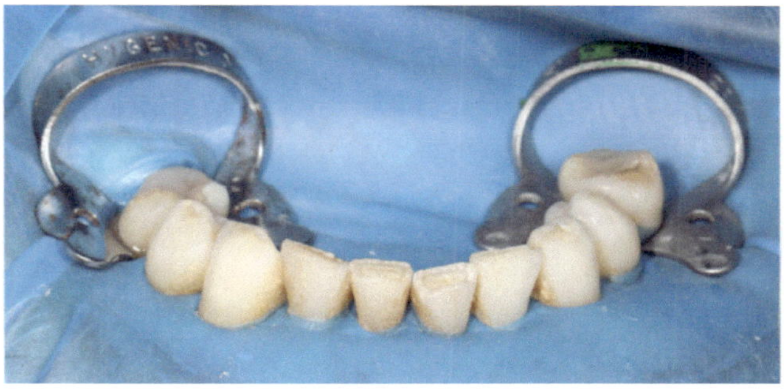

FIGURE 122

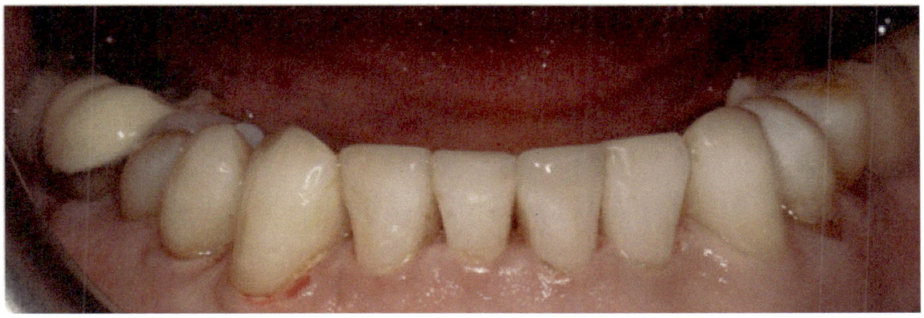

Below you can see the upper arch for the same patient. Once more because I'm building palatally my floss ties are on the buccal. This is because I don't want to incorporate them into the composite. ***Figure 123*** shows the isolation, and ***Figure 124*** shows the finished build up.

FIGURE 123

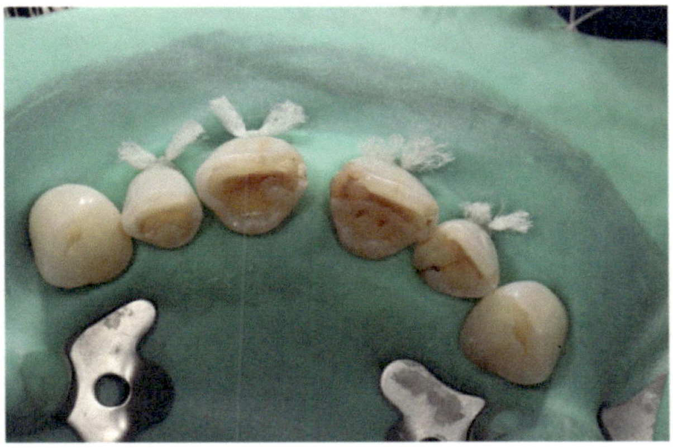

FIGURE 124

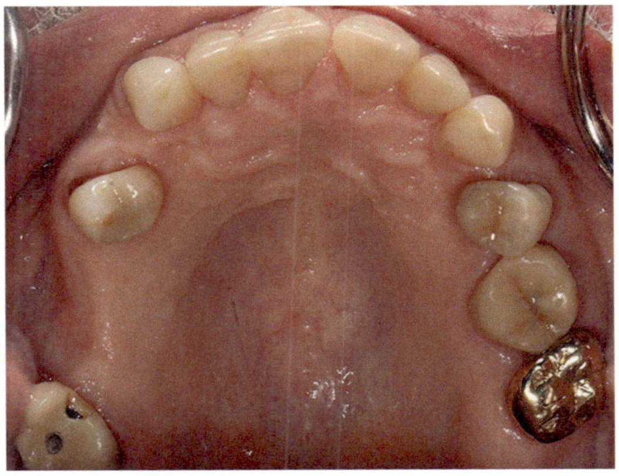

I am using the same protocol repeatedly. It is very predictable, so this is the protocol I use for all my bonding cases when I'm building them up. However, as I said there are other methods available.

Figure 125 shows finished treatment from the anterior view. The patient was not keen on aesthetics as he was 86 years old and did not want building upper incisal edges and wanted to keep the diastema.

FIGURE 125

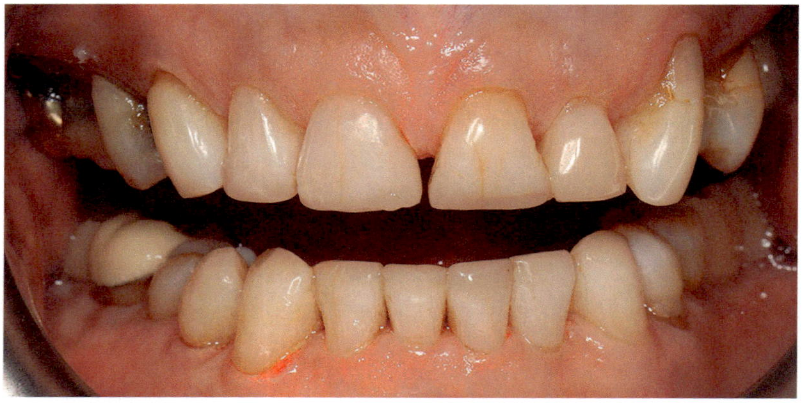

Direct build up

Let's look at another two techniques for direct build up.

- One of them is **Injection moulding**
  Injection moulding is helpful when you are building the anterior buccal. If you know you're doing direct buccal veneer then this technique is really helpful. However, you need to be very careful using this technique if you're doing buccal palatal and incisal build up. In my professional opinion it involves a lot and you need a lot of expertise to do this technique. I am also not sure if the material is meant for such a large build up at once due to more shrinkage and wear properties.

- The other technique which has been popularised in the UK is called the **Smilefast Technique**
  Smilefast Technique uses heated composite, stents are placed to provide guidance when everything is pressed onto the teeth and everything is built up in one go. This technique requires a lot more polishing, trimming and so forth. This is why the technique I have demonstrated to you when I'm building the teeth is **a better choice in my professional opinion**.

So once you have built the teeth up, next you are going to check the occlusion.

Figure 126 illustrates assessing protrusive and lateral guidance.

FIGURE 126

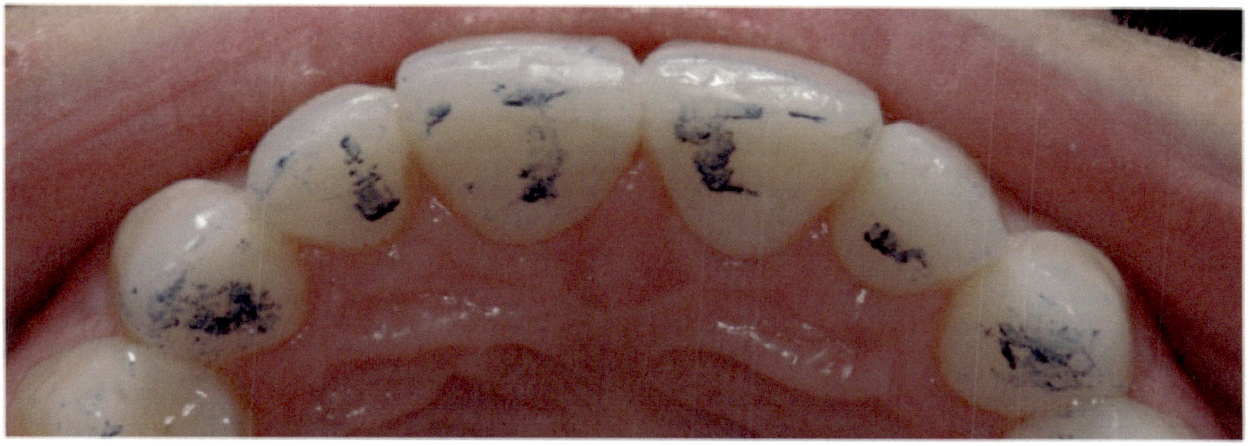

Make sure that you have protrusive guidance using two or more teeth, you have achieved your lateral guidance using canine guidance. If canine guidance is not possible then I would suggest you build premolars to make sure at the end of the appointment you have lateral guidance. It is not ideal to have lateral guidance on lateral or central incisors.

Stabilising posteriors

Now you are going to stabilise the posterior teeth, because you don't want them to supra-erupt while you're waiting for your work to stabilise. It also gives posterior stability and more comfort to patients.

There are usually two methods available to you:

1. You can take indices from your wax up and make provisionals using bisacryl material. You can either shrink fit them or cement them using temporary cement.
2. I prefer to keep things simple and easy. Hence, I usually would put in some GIC Stops as shown in ***Figure 127.*** When I'm placing GIC I want to put the stops on the occlusal surface and not go beyond the marginal ridges. This is because when you take impressions for your secondary wax up, your technician can identify individual teeth and she/he doesn't have to use imagination. Often, they can simply trim that GIC out a little bit and build the teeth around it. This will also help you in seating your indices when it comes to doing posterior build up.

FIGURE 127

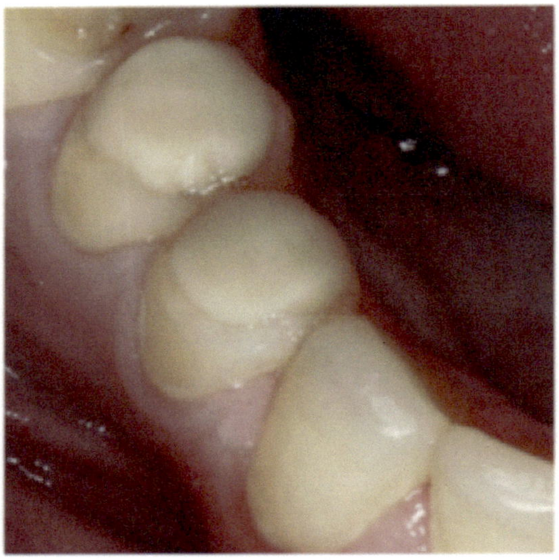

An example you can see in ***Figure 128*** is a patient who is now ready for a posterior build up. You can see the GIC stops, at the time of build up we simply remove these stops using a fast handpiece and use indices taken from our second way up to build posterior teeth using stamp technique (discussed in Step 3 of the process). You can see in this picture I have removed GIC stops from LL4 and LL6 and the patient is now ready for the build up of those two teeth.

FIGURE 128

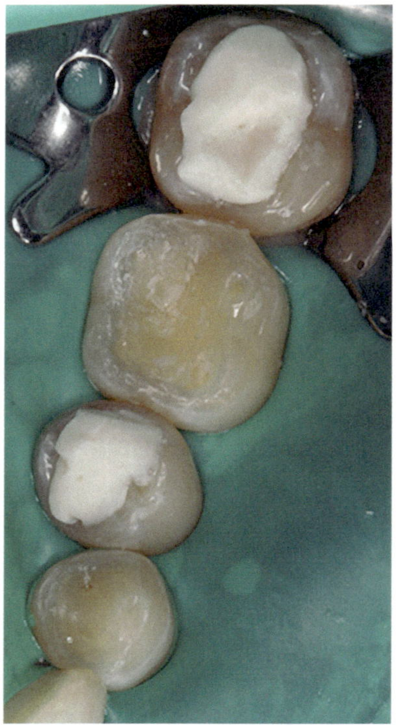

It's very easy to use GIC. You just place GIC on the tooth on either upper or lower arch, usually doing a couple of teeth at a time. You apply some Vaseline/petroleum jelly on the opposing arch and ask the patient to close while the GIC is setting. Be sure to ask them to keep their mouth closed until it sets.

Now you have that stop, make sure that it is stable. GIC is made from a much better quality material nowadays and they do stay in place as long as you have followed manufacturer's guidelines.

Once you have reached this stage you are going to review your patient on a weekly or two weekly basis for up to four weeks. Make sure that everything is stable, that you and your patient are happy.

Next you are going to move on to the posterior build ups.

3.3 Anterior Indirect Restorations

In this section we will be doing a recap for the many indirect methods which are available for building anterior teeth.

You can use composite palatal backing, ceramic palatal backing, gold palatal backing or full coverage crown.

If you are doing the direct-indirect or semi direct/sandwich method, then you will build up the palatal surface and incisal length using composite. Once you have completed the full mouth reconstruction you can then change the anterior teeth into veneers while keeping the palatal composite backings.

Composite palatal backing

This book is mainly about direct full mouth reconstruction. However, we still need to discuss indirect composite backings. This is because they can be useful in cases where you have more than 2mm of build up to do and you do not feel confident in building large direct palatal backings.

In this case, you can see that the patient in ***Figure 129*** has got quite severe wear on the palatal aspect. There is almost no cingulum.

FIGURE 129

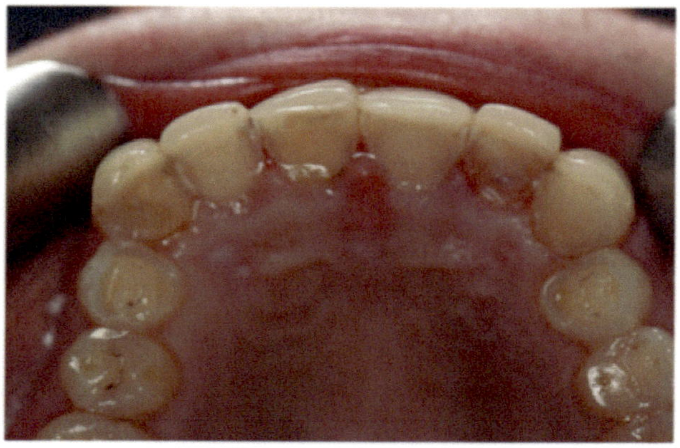

So we took the impressions, we did the wax up of the teeth (***Figure 130***) and did a trial in the patient's mouth.

FIGURE 130

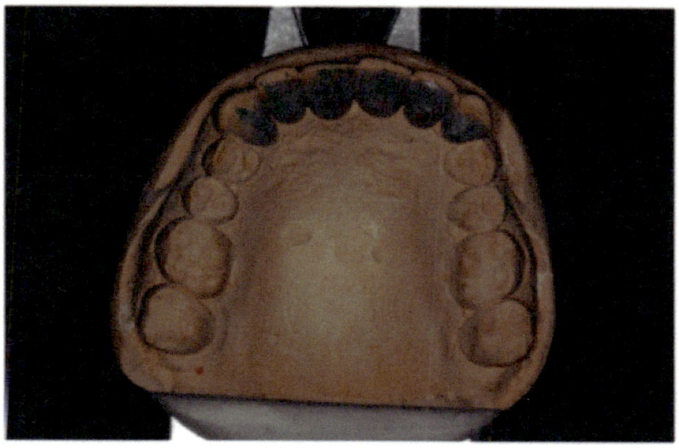

The patient was happy with the wax up so now we took new impressions (***Figure 131***). Then, we electroplated the impression (***Figure 132***) and made a model. This case including all the lab work was done by me.

FIGURE 131

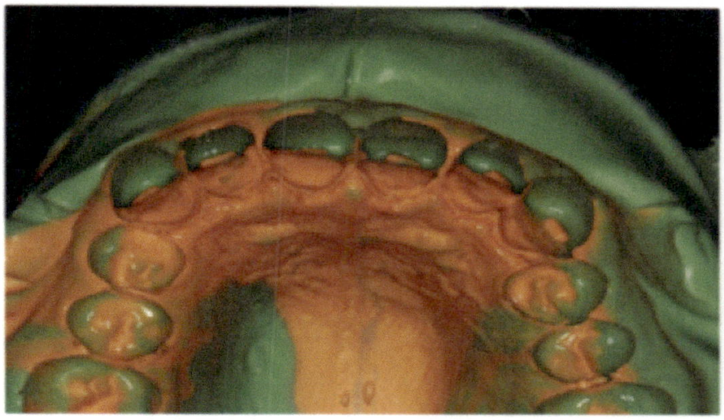

FIGURE 132

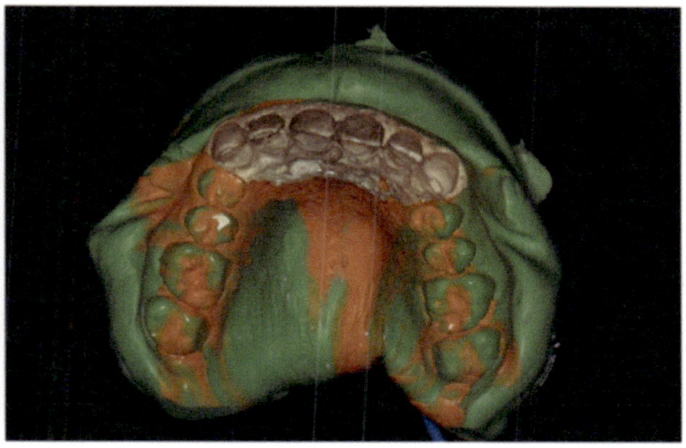

The advantage of electroplating and making a model with silver dyes is that it doesn't wear and that the fit is very accurate (***Figure 133).***

FIGURE 133

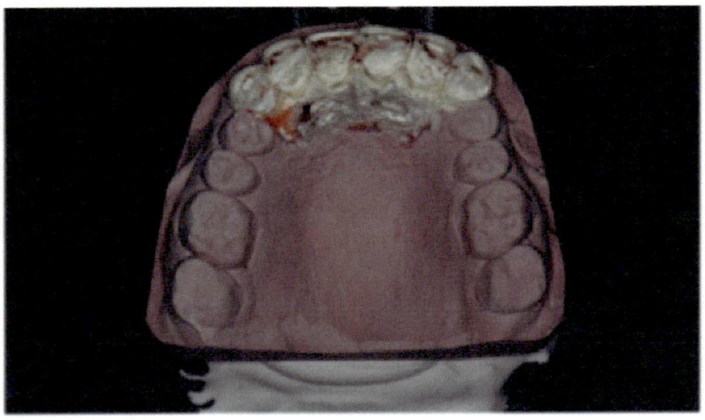

Once that was done we mounted the model on an articulator in CR (***Figure 134***). And then I went ahead and made the indirect composite backings (***Figure 135***).

FIGURE 134

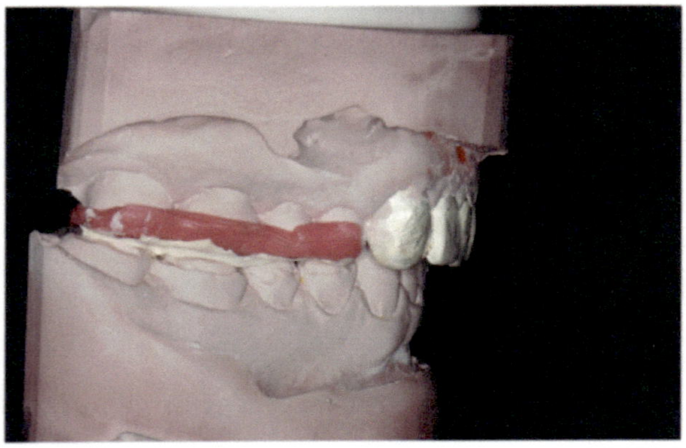

FIGURE 135

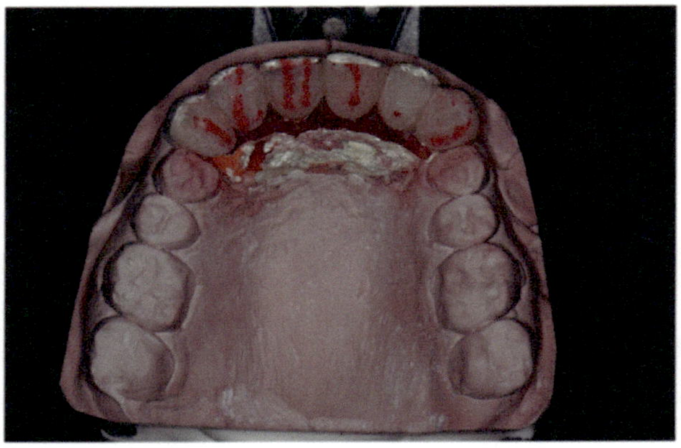

Figure 136 is when I am checking occlusion after finishing and ***Figure 137*** is me making sure it is polished – something to always remember.

FIGURE 136

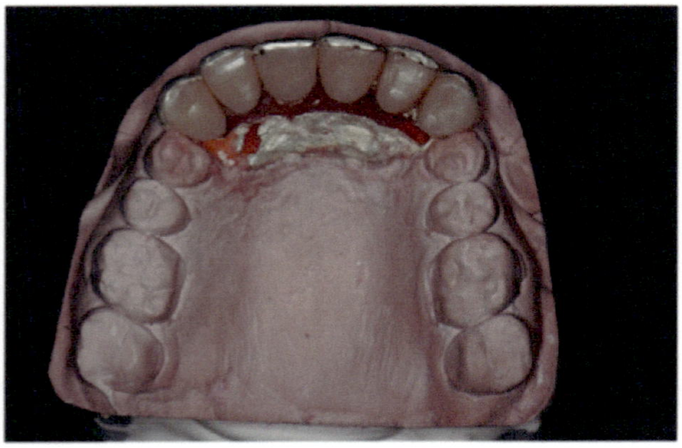

FIGURE 137

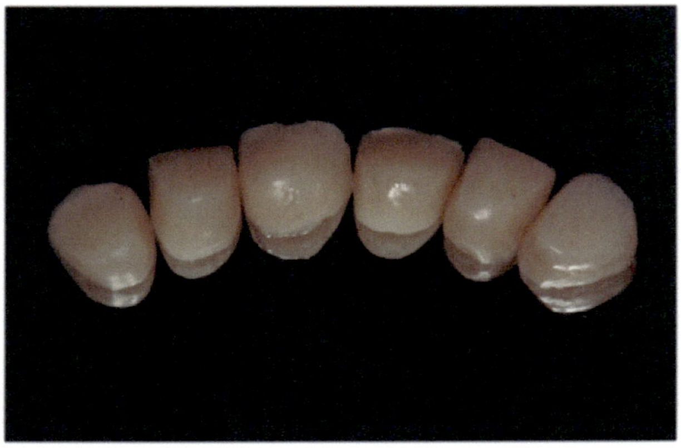

Next, I bonded the palatal backings the way you bond veneers, except it is on the palatal surface. ***Figure 138*** shows the isolation.

FIGURE 138

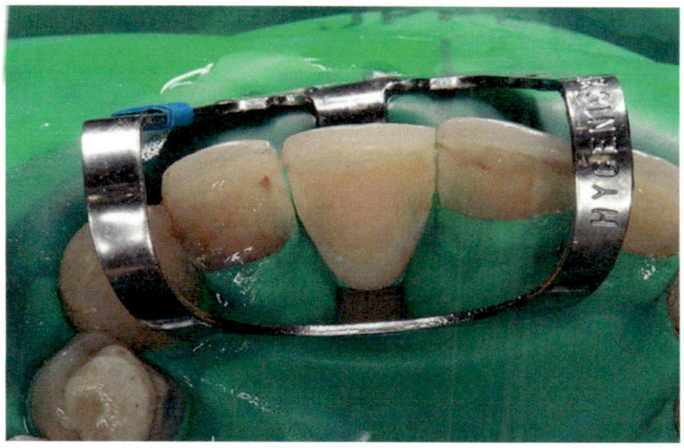

Here I followed exactly the same protocol we have discussed in detail above. Isolation, etching, bonding, priming and bonding the composite backings onto the polished surface of the teeth. Doing this one tooth at a time. ***Figure 139a*** shows the application of the bond, and ***Figure 139b*** shows finishing the first palatal backing bonding.

FIGURE 139a

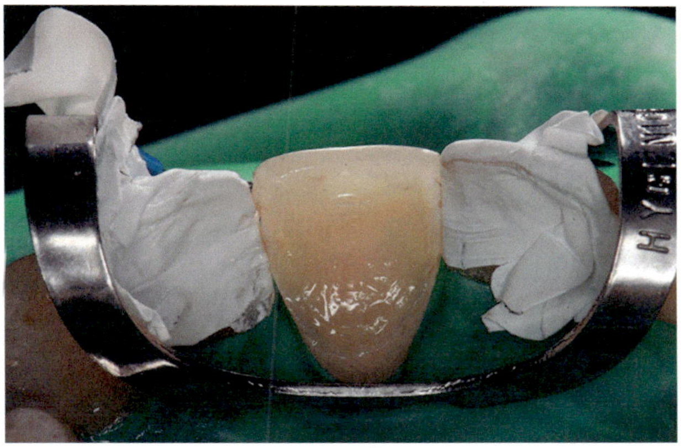

FIGURE 139b

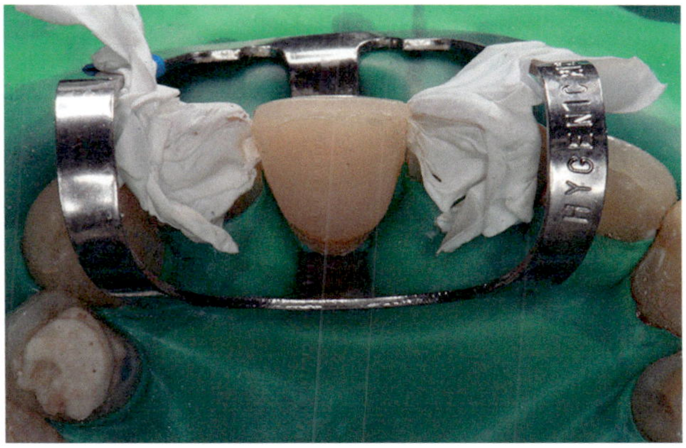

Here are the end results on the day of the treatment. As you can see in ***Figure 140a*** which shows the finished result, and ***Figure 140b*** shows assessment of occlusion.

FIGURE 140a

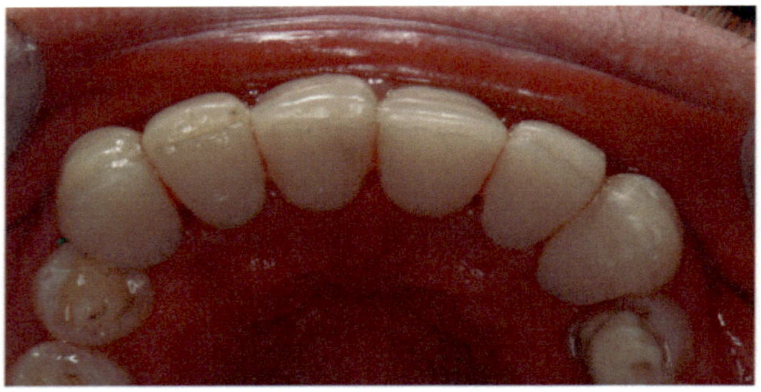

FIGURE 140b

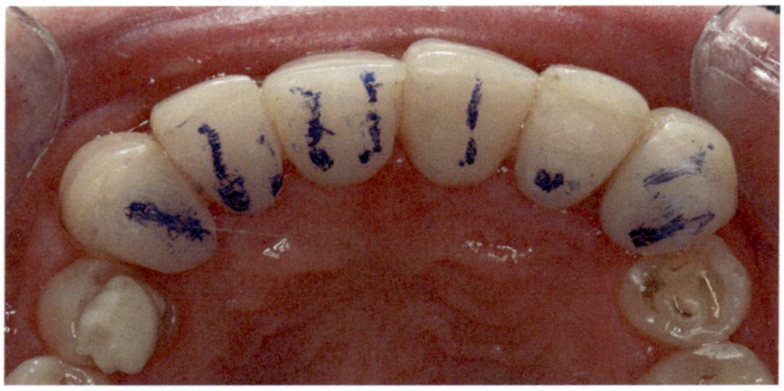

The patient had no issues whatsoever because we tested everything. We tested when doing the mock-up and made sure the patient was satisfied with the mock up before proceeding. The other option would have been to do orthodontic treatment. The problem was the patient had already received orthodontic treatment and there was a sign of root absorption. So, this was a compromise case. However, I have only included it to show you how to do indirect palatal backings and how to bond them.

If your patient has severe buccal, incisal and palatal wear, then you need to consider full coverage restoration or sandwich technique. These are the preparations which can be done with minimal invasiveness if you are building a whole tooth and space has already been created due to pre-existing wear.

As discussed above, after anterior reconstruction you will need to make sure you have stabilised the posterior teeth. This is to give your patient more comfort during the transition period, to enable stability while mounting models and to prevent any movement of the teeth.

Now that the patient's anterior teeth are built and you have reviewed the patient and everything looks fine then you are ready to move to the step 3 of the process which is building posterior teeth.

CHAPTER 4

Step 3: Posterior Reconstruction

4.1 Posterior Direct Build-Up

In this section we are going to discuss posterior build-up.

Previously, we've done anterior build-up, we have stabilised the posterior teeth using GIC stops or with possible temporaries using diagnostic wax up.

We assess our patient between one and two weeks after, in order to assess occlusion, occlusal stops and to make sure everything is stable. During these assessments we complete any necessary refinement.

Now we are at this stage of the journey shown in ***Figure 141a*** and ***Figure 141b*** where we build anterior teeth and the posterior teeth are not in contact.

FIGURE 141a

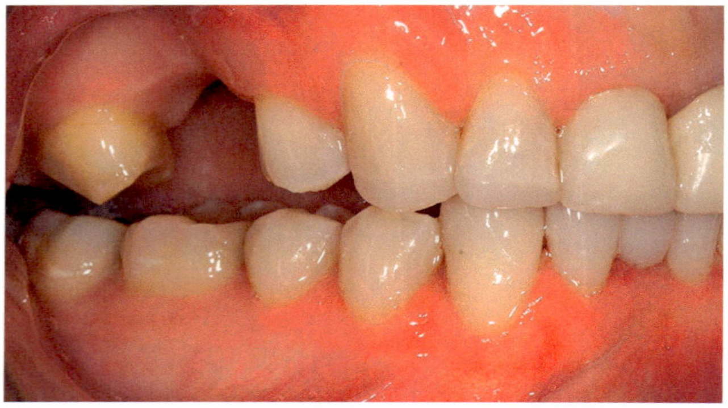

FIGURE 141b

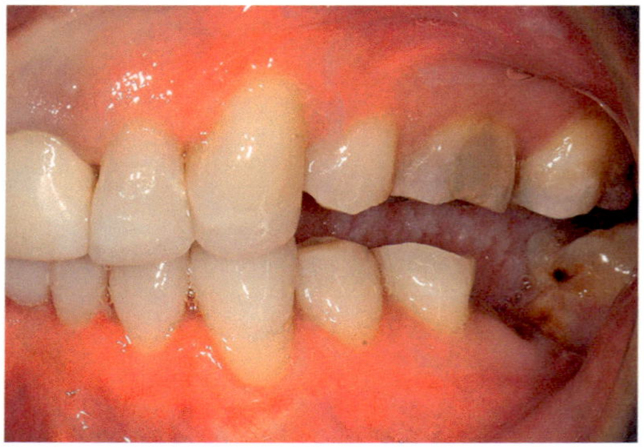

Now I am going to show you how to reach the step shown in ***Figure 141c*** and ***Figure 141d.*** We are at the stage where we are building the posterior teeth with direct or indirect restoration. We are creating the occlusion or the bite we need in order to complete our full mouth reconstruction.

FIGURE 141c

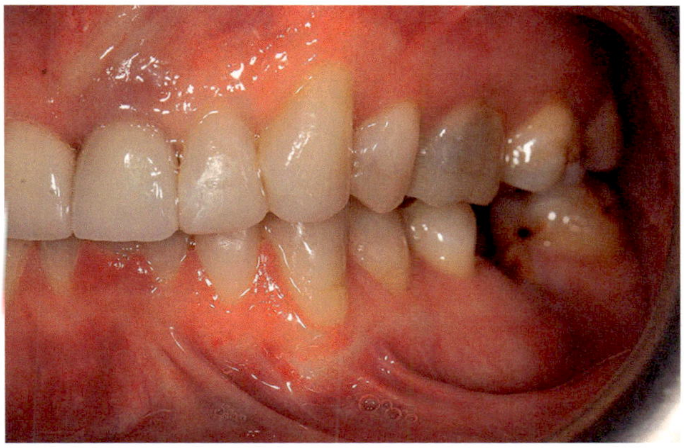

FIGURE 141d

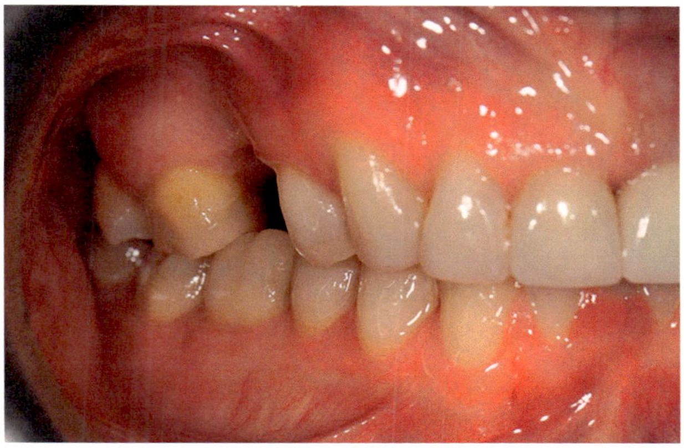

New records in ICP

After completing anterior build up, you need to take new impressions.

- **Take upper and lower impressions + facebow + Bite reg in ICP.**
  We need to take upper and lower putty and wash impressions. We need to take facebow. You don't need to do a lucia jig and make a CR record because your anterior six teeth are in ICP which is same as CO. All we need to do now is take ICP records. You do not need to remove the GIC stops.

  When recording interocclusal bite in ICP, you need to place the bite registration material between posterior teeth and simply ask your patient to close their teeth. Then technician will articulate models in ICP. The technician will use facebow to mount the model on the semi-adjustable articulator, or arbitrary, or average value articulator. Then the lower model will be mounted using the bite registration material we provided in ICP. Because we already have our patient in CO and the position is ideal, CO will equal ICP, making this a much more relaxed position.

  I advise sending your lab all the information you have for mounting and make sure you describe to the lab exactly what you want them to do. Do not be shy in giving detailed instructions.

4.2 Steps in Posterior Direct Build-Up

Once models are mounted, there are two requirements you may find very useful to advise your laboratory of:

1. You can advise your laboratory to wax up alternative teeth, to duplicate the model and continue waxing the remaining teeth.
2. If you are doing indirect restorations then make sure you do the direct restorations first. You have much more control once the direct restorations are done. You have the shape of the teeth and occlusion is right and your technician just needs to use that as a baseline when they are fabricating the indirect restorations.

So if you are doing a combination of direct and indirect restorations for posterior teeth, then the direct restoration will be waxed up first. The reason we do alternative teeth wax up is that when you are creating indices, you want either side of the tooth as a stop. You don't want them to be waxed up otherwise your indices will have no support to be stable because the index is not sitting properly on the patient's teeth as all the teeth have been waxed up.

Alternative tooth wax up

Here is an example wax up for reference. We are building the first premolar, first molar and second molar on both sides. We are not building the third molar and hence it does not need wax up. We are building 3 posterior teeth per side.

You can see on ***Figure 142a*** that alternative teeth are waxed up. To demonstrate two different methods, I have waxed up two teeth on one side and one tooth on the other. However, it does not matter as long as the tooth next to the waxed up tooth is not altered with wax. Once this wax up is done then your technician will duplicate the model which you can use to make your first set of indices. The technician will carry on waxing up the rest of the teeth. You can see this on ***Figure 142b***.

FIGURE 142a

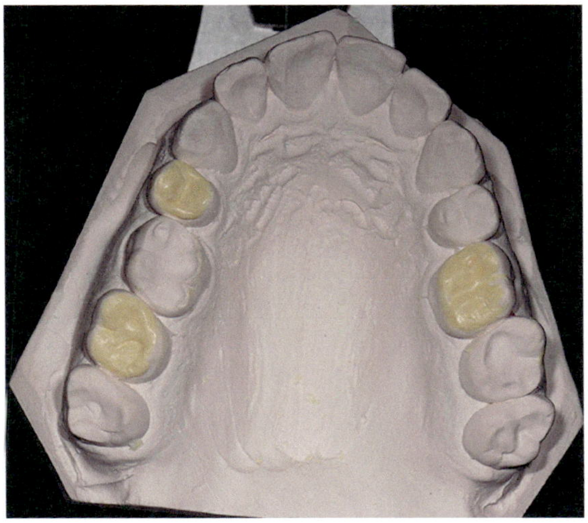

FIGURE 142b

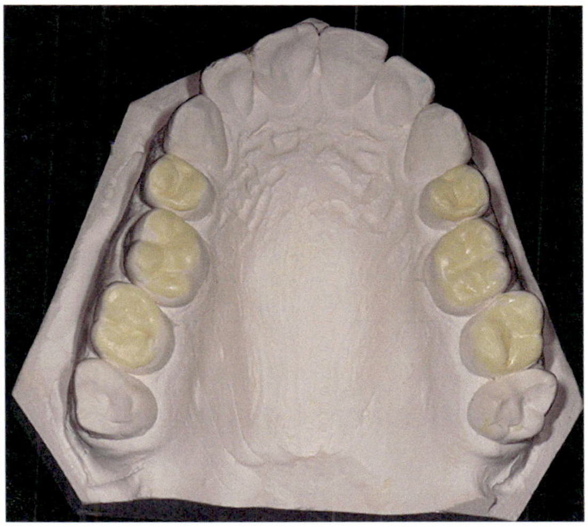

Here you can see the same process with the lower jaw. In ***Figure 143a*** we're doing wax up of alternative teeth, duplicating the model and then waxing up the remaining the teeth in ***Figure 143b***.

FIGURE 143a

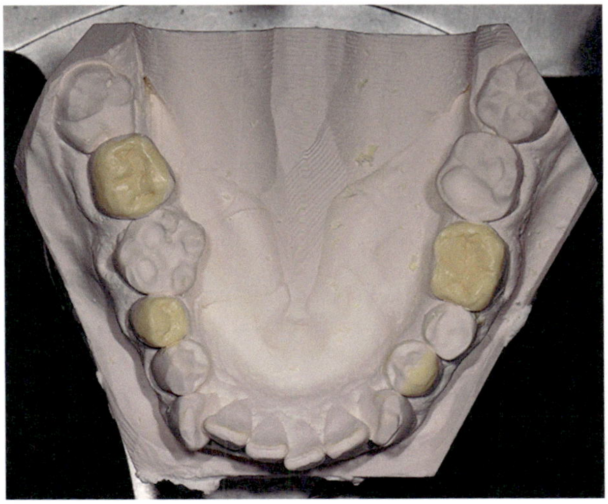

FIGURE 143b

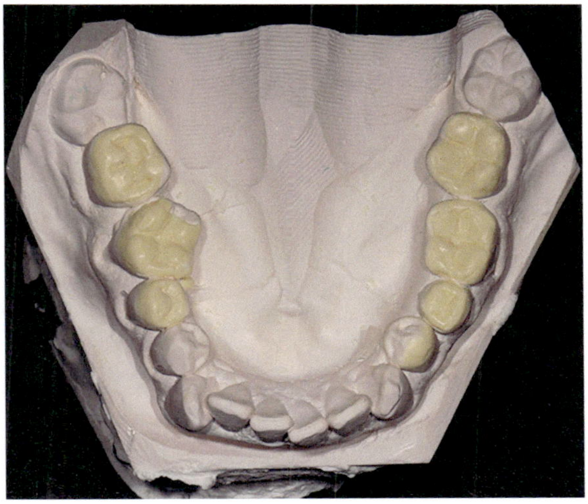

4.3 Techniques

In this chapter we look at the methods you can use to build posterior teeth up. You can use a direct restoration method or indirect restoration method.

Within **Direct Restorations** you can have:

- Stamp method (Exaclear/Memosil).
- Putty index.
- Direct freehand build up.

Within **Indirect Restorations** you can have:

- Onlays (Lithium disilicate, Composite, Hybrid, Gold).
- Crowns (Lithium disilicate, Zirconia, Gold).

In this chapter we're going to concentrate on the direct build up of the teeth.

Using clear stent (stamp technique)

Let's look at the first technique where we're using Exaclear stent for the direct technique. In ***Figures 144*** and ***145*** you can see both the Exaclear and the model.

This model is to be used for my second index. I will be using an alternative tooth wax up model for my first set of indices. I'm going to use the alternative tooth model to take the index of the alternative teeth.

FIGURE 144

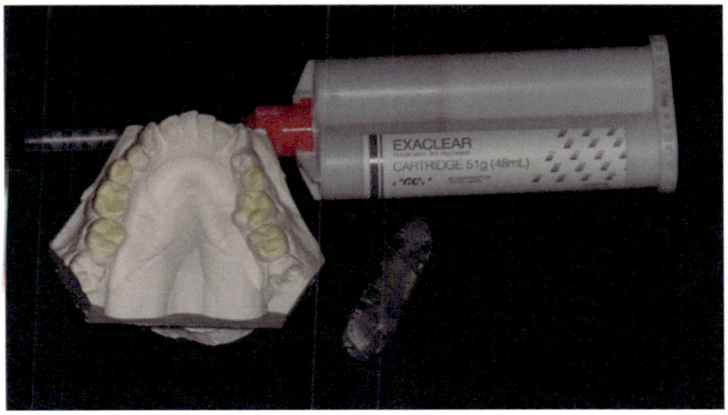

FIGURE 145

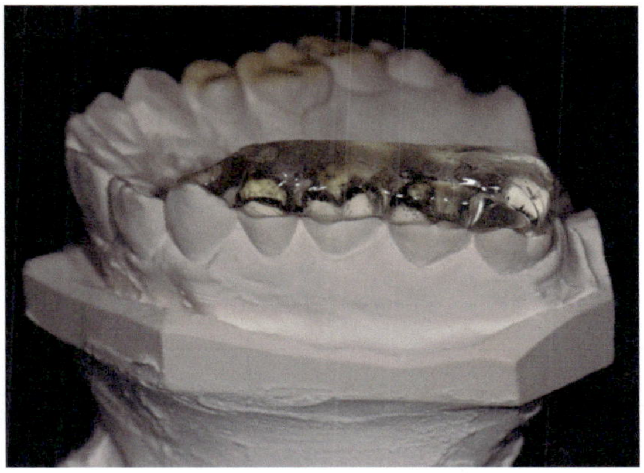

You can see in ***Figure 146*** and ***Figure 147*** the teeth that we are planning to build clinically.

FIGURE 146

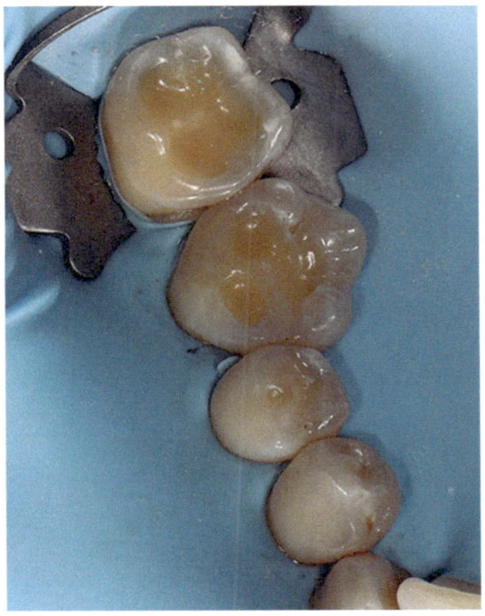

FIGURE 147

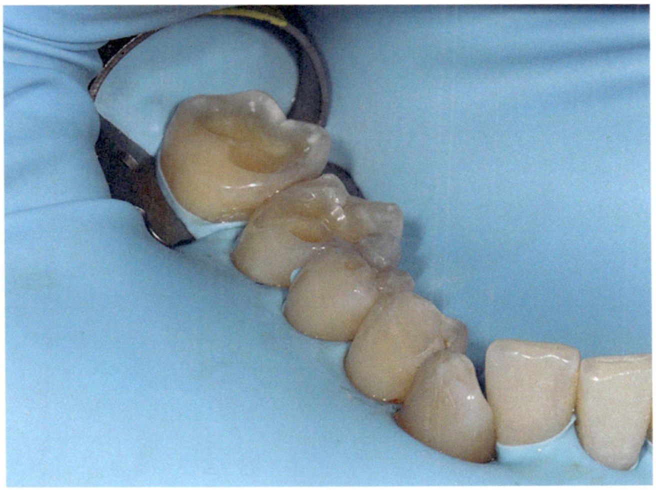

In ***Figure 148*** I'm checking the fit of my index. This index is taken from the model where we did alternative tooth wax up.

FIGURE 148

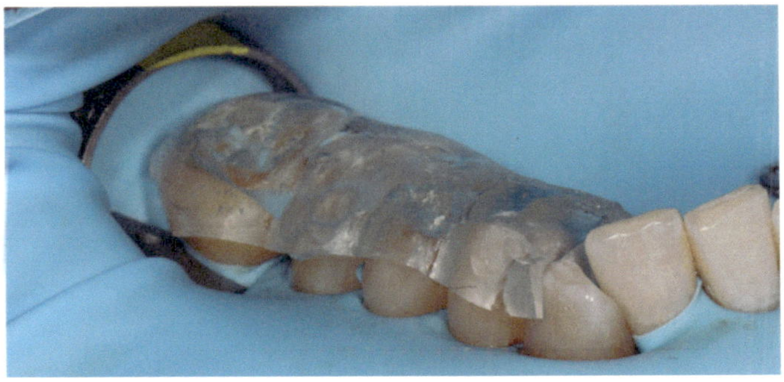

Once we have trimmed and made sure the teeth are the way we want them, we can etch, prime and bond alternative teeth after isolating neighboring teeth with PTFE tape**.** Then load heated composite onto the indices and place some on the tooth and press the index on the tooth, keep pressing the index until its completely seated. You can see in ***Figure 149*** that I have bonded and built up the second premolar and second molar.

Now I use the index made from the model where all the teeth were waxed up. In ***Figure 150*** I'm checking the fit of that index.

FIGURE 149

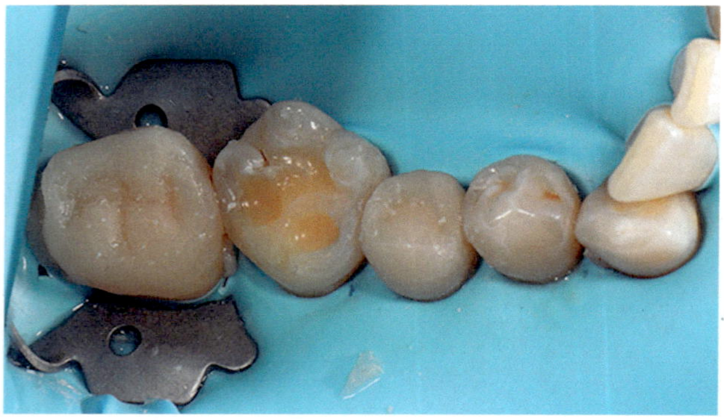

FIGURE 150

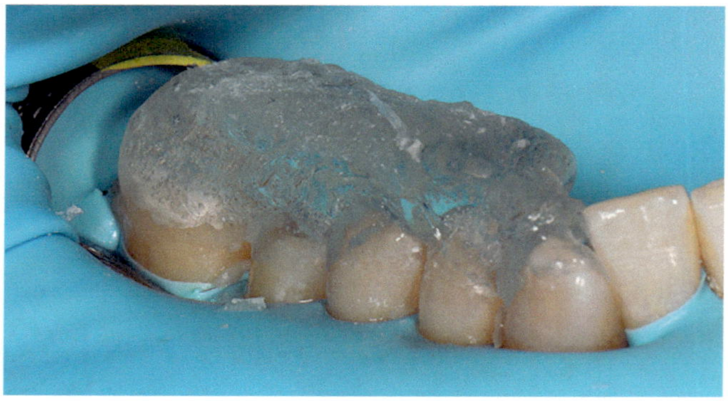

As shown in ***Figure 151a***, cover everything on both sides of the teeth with PTFE and squash heated composite. Then use a stamp technique to create the desired anatomy. ***Figure 151b*** shows the tooth just after removal of the index. This is a very easy and effective way to build teeth.

FIGURE 151a

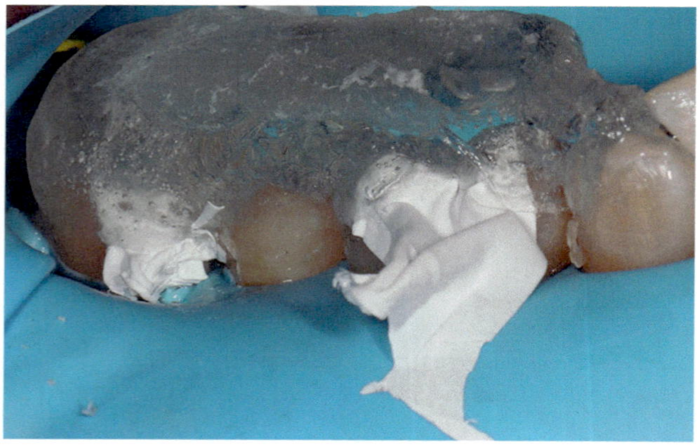

FIGURE 151b

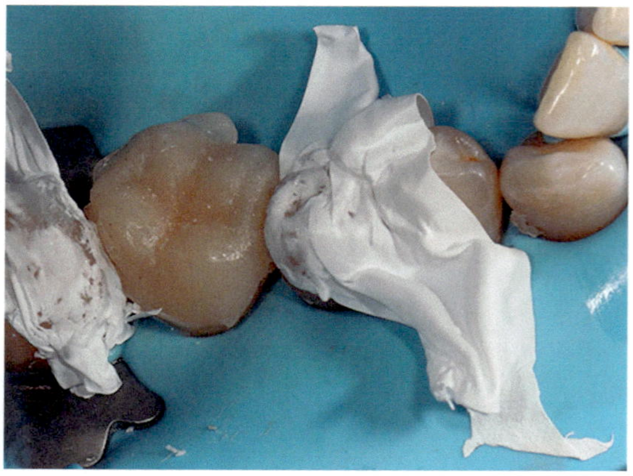

Result after polishing shown in ***Figure 152*** and ***Figure 153.***

FIGURE 152

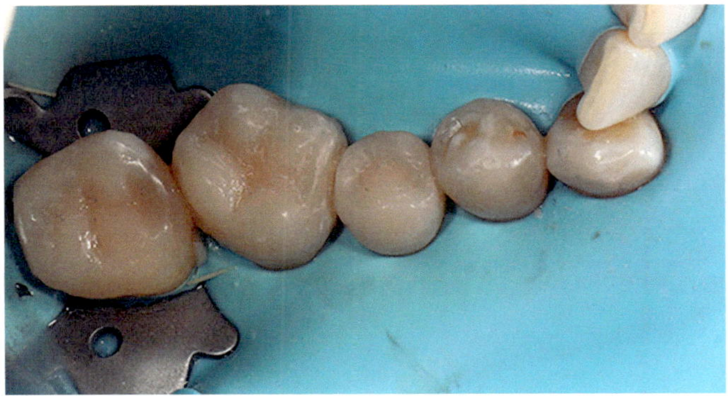

FIGURE 153

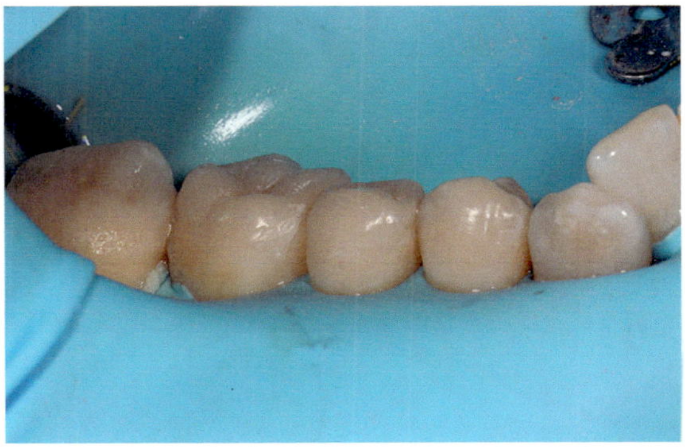

After doing one side, I follow the same procedure with the other teeth (***Figure 154***). Next we check the indices to make sure the fit is good (***Figure 155***).

FIGURE 154

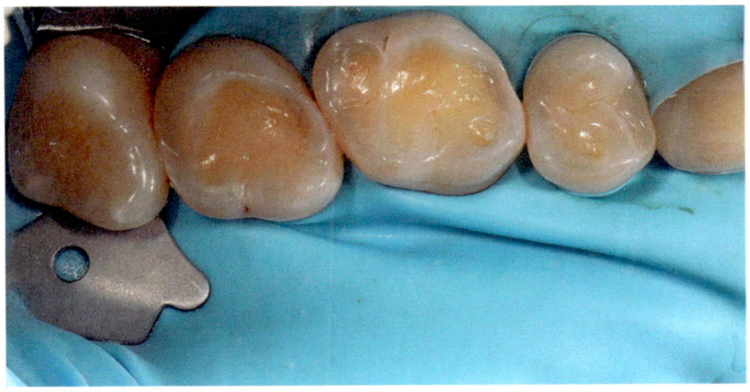

FIGURE 155

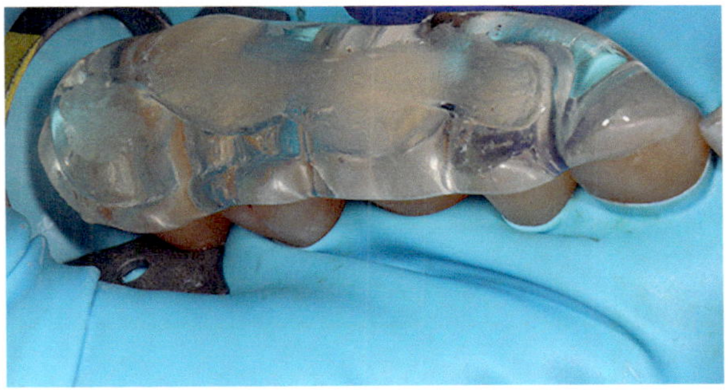

Then we build up alternative teeth ***Figure 156***.

FIGURE 156

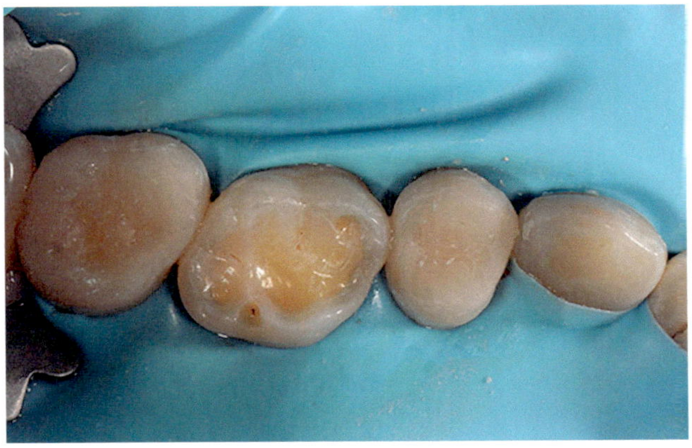

Lastly, we do the remaining tooth at the end. All this is done using the stamp technique. It is a very quick and efficient way to do the posterior build up, especially for teeth which are not filled and just need build up.

If you have teeth which have large old restorations then it is advisable to remove those old restorations. Make sure to remove caries and restore teeth with composite to original shape before you take an impression for a wax up. This will make your work much easier when it comes to doing occlusal build ups as all you will be doing is building the occlusal table.

In ***Figure 157a*** I am checking the first for the next index, in ***Figure 157b*** I am isolating with PTFE.

FIGURE 157a

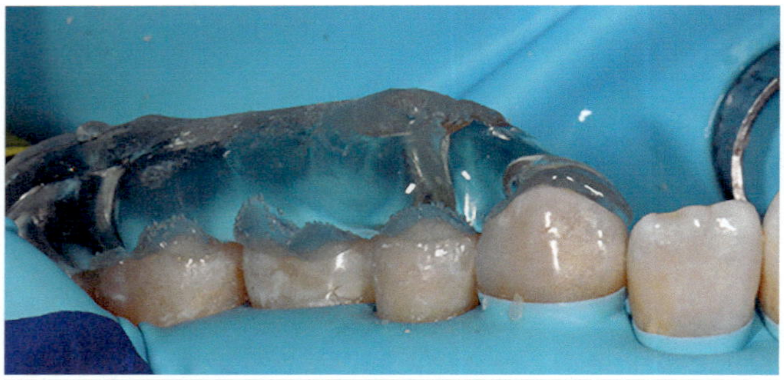

FIGURE 157b

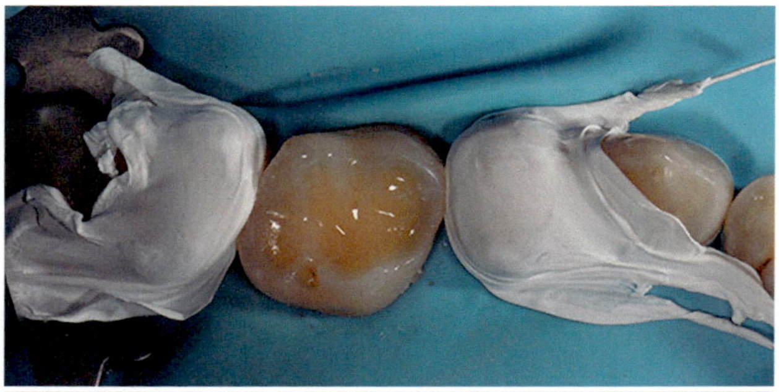

In ***Figure 157c*** I am placing the index with composite. ***Figure 157d*** shows the tooth after the removal of the composite, ***Figure 157e*** shows finished result, ***Figures 157f*** and ***157g*** illustrate assessing the occlusion.

FIGURE 157c

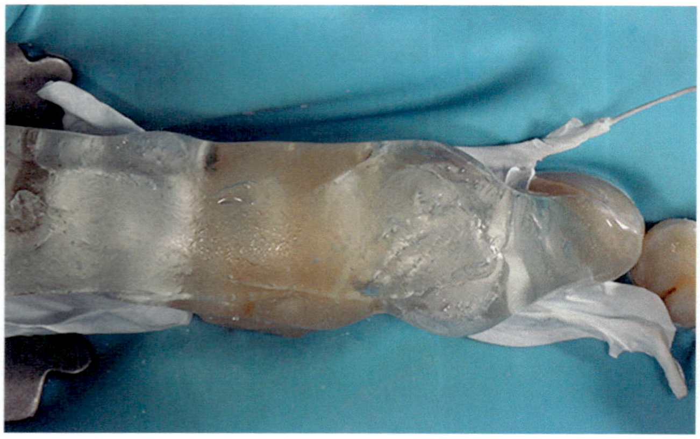

FIGURE 157d

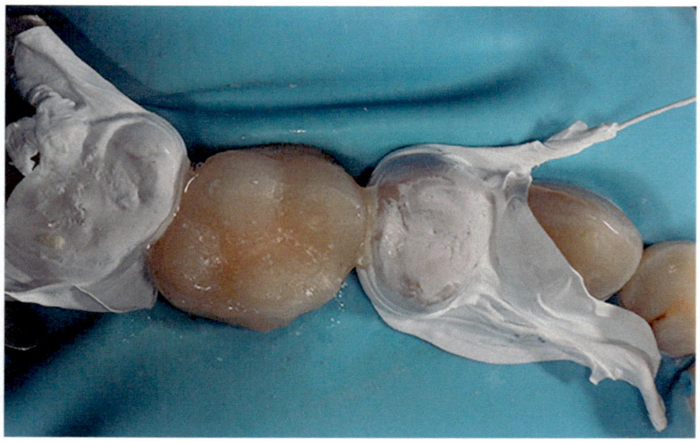

FIGURE 157e

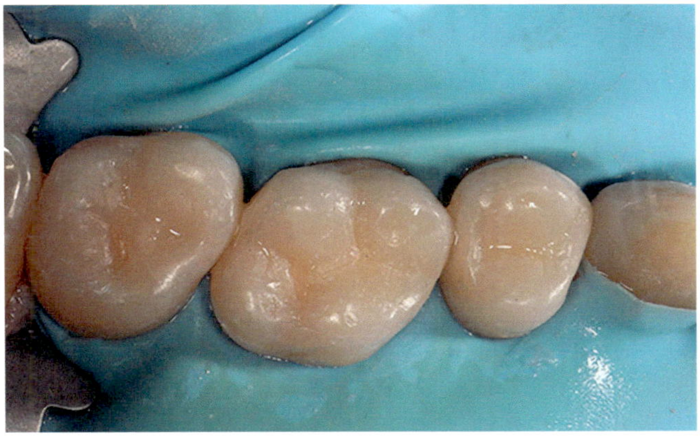

Once the build up is completed, we need to check occlusion for ICP contacts, making sure that there is no non working side contact nor there is any unplanned guidance.

FIGURE 157f

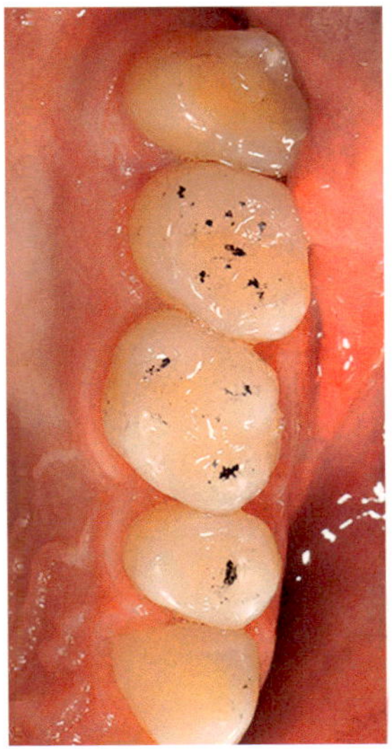

FIGURE 157g

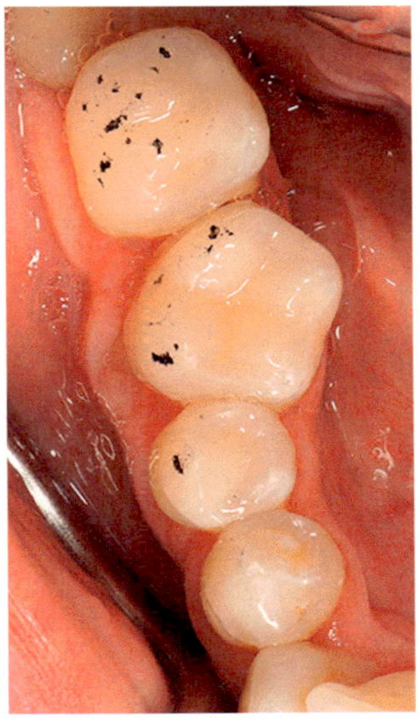

Putty index technique

This is my back up technique for posterior teeth. The reason I first used this technique is that I went to a practice to mentor someone and they did not have Exaclear. So I had to improvise for the case in ***Figure 158***.

FIGURE 158

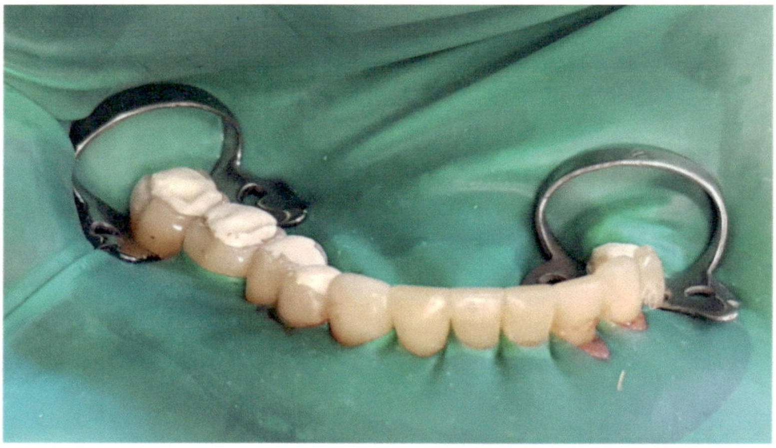

We used putty indices. You cut the putty from the buccal cusp tip and this is what you see in ***Figure 159.*** Then what you do is push the composite from the buccal area and build the teeth. As you can see in ***Figure 160*** this technique gave acceptable results.

FIGURE 159

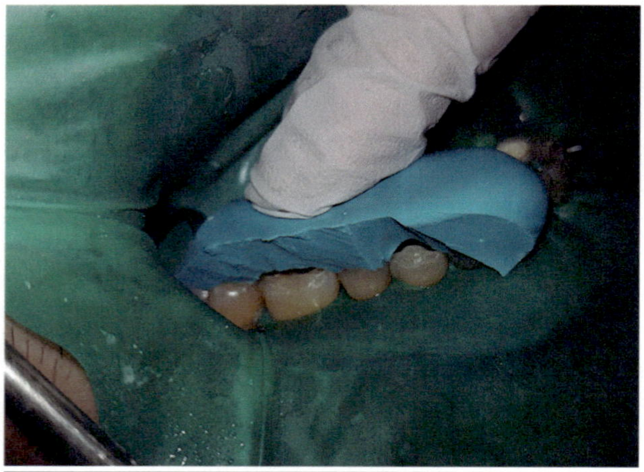

FIGURE 160

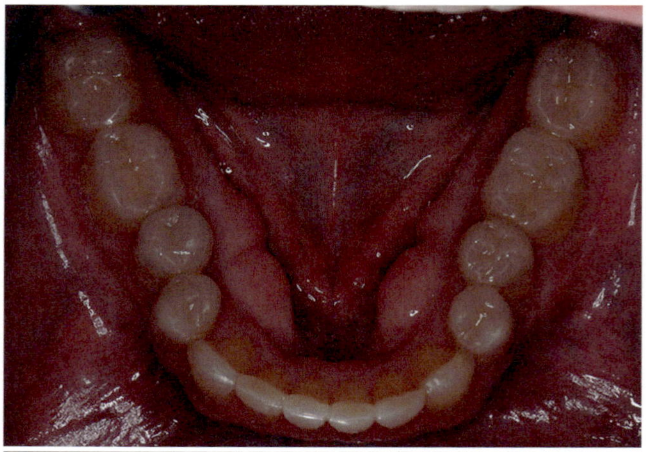

Having said that, the procedure is significantly easier if you use Exaclear, so I advise doing so whenever possible.

Freehand technique

The other method is freehand technique. The patient in ***Figure 161a*** and ***Figure 161b*** was anteriorly done using stamp technique. However, the posterior reconstruction involved only minor additions so I did it using the freehand technique.

FIGURE 161a

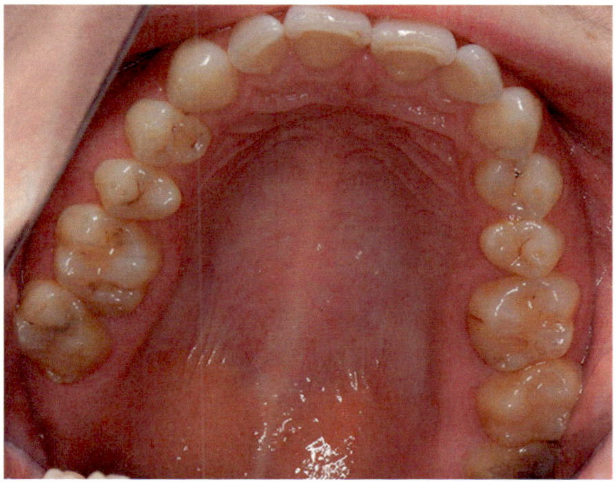

FIGURE 161b

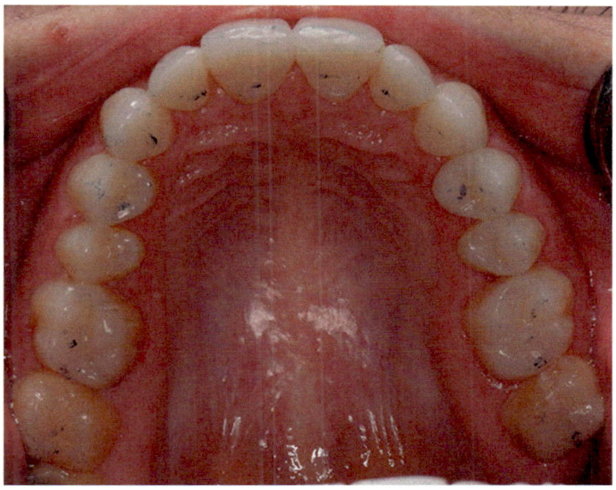

After posterior reconstruction, checking the occlusion is vital. Once you finish the posterior reconstruction, check the occlusion. Make sure the anterior occlusion, protrusive and lateral guidance is the way you planned it (***Figure 162***). Make sure there are no interferences between the posterior teeth, check the contact points, and make sure you haven't lost any contact points. Do the same assessment you do for Michigan splint after you finish your posterior reconstruction.

FIGURE 162

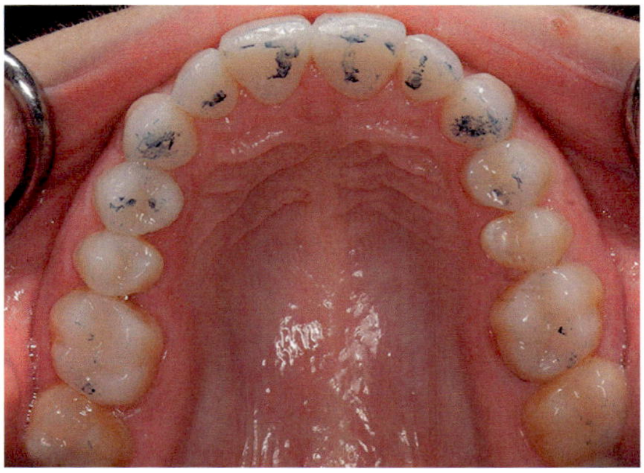

In the next chapter, we are going to review maintenance and protection for full mouth reconstruction patients.

CHAPTER 5

Maintenance and Protection

In this chapter we are going to discuss the maintenance of full mouth reconstruction patients.

So far we have discussed three steps. Step number 1 - treatment planning, step number 2 - anterior buildup, step number 3 - posterior buildup.

When it comes to doing maintenance, I would break it down into three aspects: **protection, hygiene and regular checkups.**

5.1 Protection

Protection is very important because if your patient has damaged their teeth by bruxism or wear there is a chance that the same thing may happen again. This is especially true for patients with bruxism or parafunctional habits.

Michigan splint

The best way to protect our restoration is with a Michigan splint (***Figure 163***). The Michigan splint, as we know from earlier in this text, is one of the best ways to relax your patient's muscles and protect their teeth at the same time.

FIGURE 163

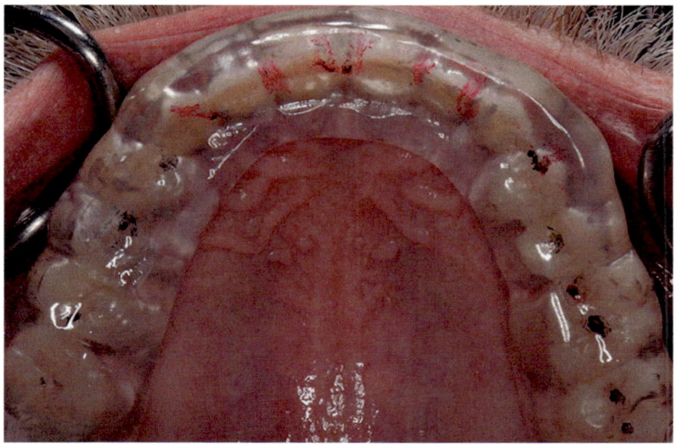

Soft night guard

However, sometimes a patient has erosive wear and there is no sign of bruxism. In such a case, you could give patients a soft night guard. A problem with this is there is some research suggesting that the soft night guard can increase the bruxism habit because it gives patients something to chew on and the patient keeps chewing that at nighttime. So I'm not a very great fan of soft night guards. However, if the patient cannot use a hard acrylic mouth guard then this option is better than nothing.

Essix retainer

If a patient has had orthodontic treatment, then you can give them an Essix retainer for the upper and lower jaw. This will also protect restoration. Alternatively, you can give them a dual arch B splint if they have any TMJ issues.

Whether this is the best option depends on the quality of the retainer and the bite of the patient. They might chew through the Essix retainer quickly and you need to be able to communicate this to your patient. They will have to pay appropriate attention and take appropriate care of the retainer. They may have to get the retainer replaced every year in some cases.

5.2 Maintenance

Hygiene

Make sure your patients are visiting a hygienist regularly. Depending on their needs patients should visit a hygienist at intervals ranging from three to six months. It further depends on how good patients are at cleaning their teeth. Some patients just need more regular appointments. You need to plan a hygiene regime together with the patient when you put them on their maintenance regime. You need to explain to the patient as to why you think they need to see a hygienist every three, four, five or six months.

Checkup

Regular checkups are very important.

If you've done direct build up then you may need to carry out polishing of the composites and repair them as needed.

You need to assess occlusion. When you discharge a patient, that occlusion will be ideal. However, over time this can change.

So, every time a patient comes for a checkup, I'll be doing the following:

- Full occlusal assessment. I will be taking my time, booking the patient for an hour, doing full occlusal assessment and sometimes my patient may need adjustment because their bite has changed a bit. I would do a full occlusal assessment.
- Assessing occlusal contacts.
- Taking appropriate radiographs, bitewings, PA's, OPG's, and anything else that needs doing.

Don't be discouraged if your patient comes back in six months or a year's time and the occlusion has changed. It has been proven that occlusion is dynamic and it keeps changing. In the 1960s people have done full mouth reconstructions just to get rid of CO to ICP slide. But it was found on a review appointment that the slide had come back.

So, occlusion changes but you need to make sure you keep checking it especially if you've done any implant restorations. Many times, when you have done implant restoration along with full mouth reconstruction and you have made sure that the implants are not heavily loaded. Patients may come back in six months' or a year's time, then their condyles may have shifted or seated properly, or they may have differential wear and they may start loading those implants more heavily. If you check the occlusion regularly then you will know of this problem before it appears.

So make sure that you do full mouth assessment including occlusal assessment and don't be worried if adjustment is needed. Make sure to let patients know of this possibility in advance as well.

Next, I have included a chapter on communication. Although you will get my communication course as a free gift when you enroll into the Practical guide to Full Mouth Reconstruction Book course, I understand that some of you may prefer to read, hence I have included some tips on communication here as well. So let us look at some of the main aspects of communication in the next chapter.

CHAPTER 6

Communication with Patients for Full Mouth Reconstruction

Communication is the key to success in any field and this field is no different. In this final chapter, we are going to discuss how best to communicate with patients about full mouth reconstruction to create winning situations.

How are full mouth reconstruction cases different to single composites or a crown?

- Full mouth reconstruction usually involves comprehensive cases.
- It involves a longer treatment plan.
- It involves higher fees.
- On many occasions you will feel some uncertainty before you start the treatment. This is because you will need to do some further investigation in order to plan the treatment properly, such as doing a diagnostic wax up or removing old restorations or crowns, before you can give the patient an idea of the exact treatment plan.
- It gets complicated with underconfident dentists who are only used to doing single tooth dentistry, and this can show when you're communicating with a patient.

Having said that, the basics of communication are the same across different disciplines of dentistry.

My Routine

- Start with building a rapport with the patient, and don't be afraid to spend a long time on this if you need to.
- Once you have a solid understanding of the patient and their needs, then you can move forward with clinical examinations, diagnoses and record taking.
- Discuss the current dental situation with the patient.
- Give them options for a treatment plan.

- Discuss fees.
- Ask them questions and answer their questions.

This is a normal routine and mustn't be rushed.

After the rapport-building and clinical assessment stages, you should get a sense of whether this is an FMR case or a simple restoration. If need be, ask the patient for more time to assess their teeth, highlighting that there is a lot going on in their mouth.

You can then reschedule the appointment, seeing them one more time in order to come up with a few options. Most patients are very appreciative of this; particularly if you don't charge to see them again, including it as part of the consultation.

Tools I use for communicating with patients

- **Photography**
  Photography is the most important tool when it comes to communicating possible options (***Figure 164***).

FIGURE 164

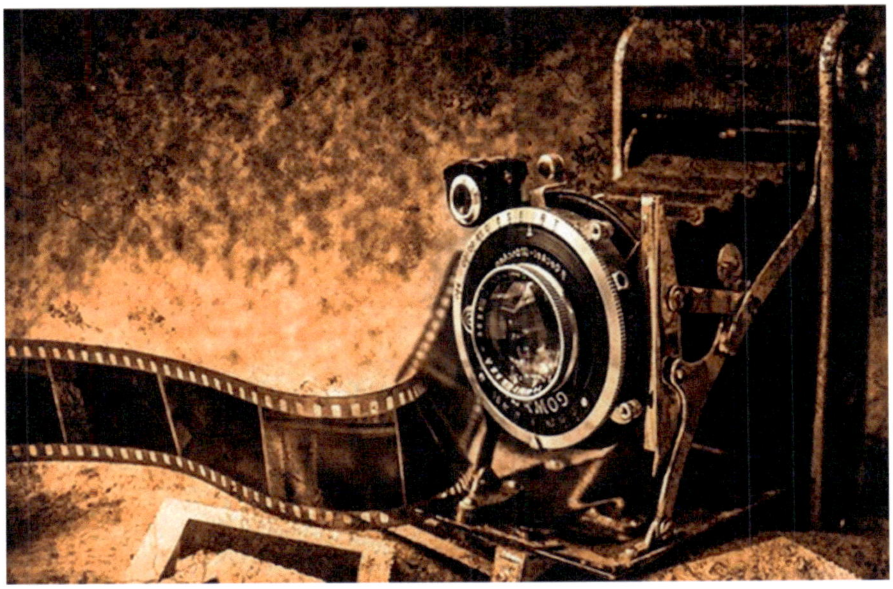

What are the different uses for photographs?

Showing caries/cracks around the tooth

Patients might object to treatment if a tooth doesn't hurt. However, taking a photo of their damaged tooth and showing it to them will mean they are less likely to contest any need for the treatment (***Figure 165***).

FIGURE 165

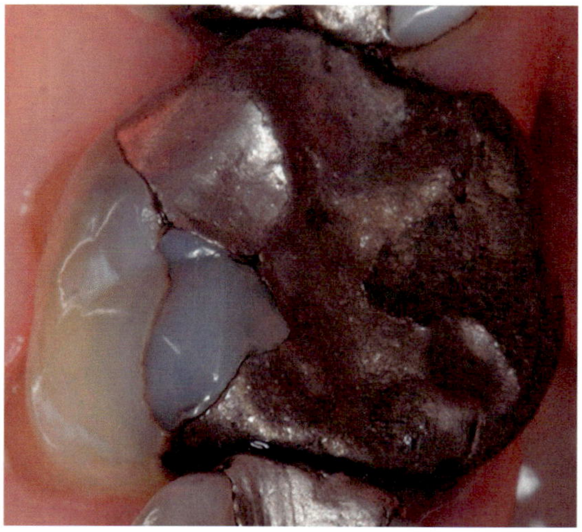

Severe caries/fracture – patient says 'can you save it'

Sometimes a patient will come to you, and ask if you can save a tooth (e.g. ***Figure 166*** shows a vertically fractured tooth). If you use photographs to show that you can't, then the patient will be likely to accept that the tooth needs to be extracted.

FIGURE 166

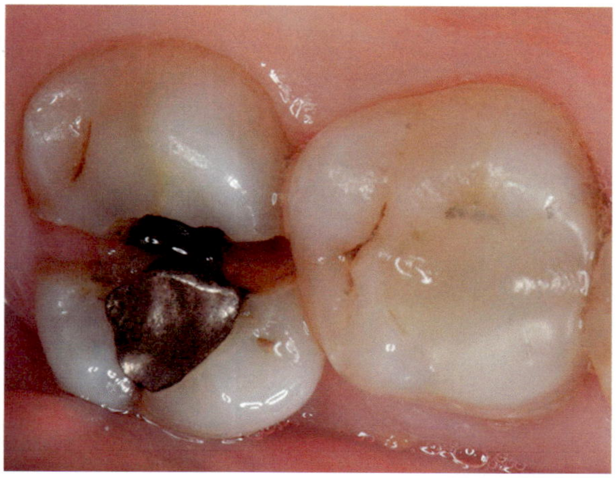

Assessment of ongoing treatment

Take a lot of photos throughout, including mid-treatment photos, to visualise and understand how things are progressing, and to communicate this to the patient.

Figure 167 shows post orthodontic treatment.

FIGURE 167a

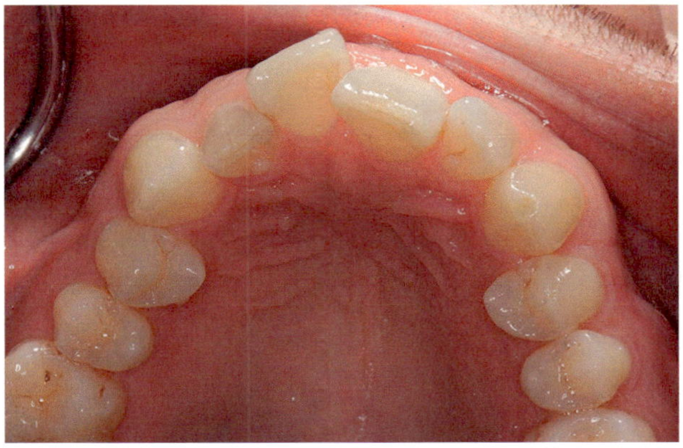

FIGURE 167b

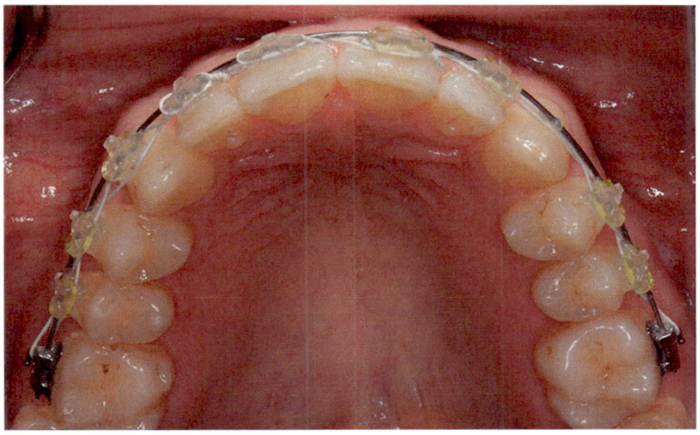

Pre treatment wax up

Photos of a study model (***Figure 168a***) and a diagnostic wax up (***Figure 168b*** and ***Figure 168c***) – mock up in the patient's mouth, or the diagnostic wax up itself, are really important.

FIGURE 168a

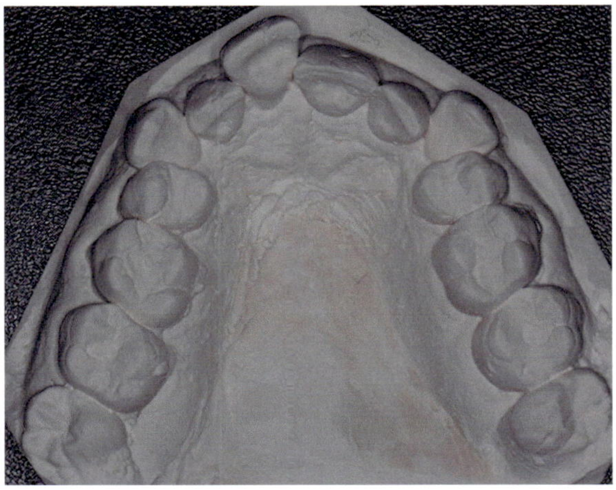

FIGURE 168b

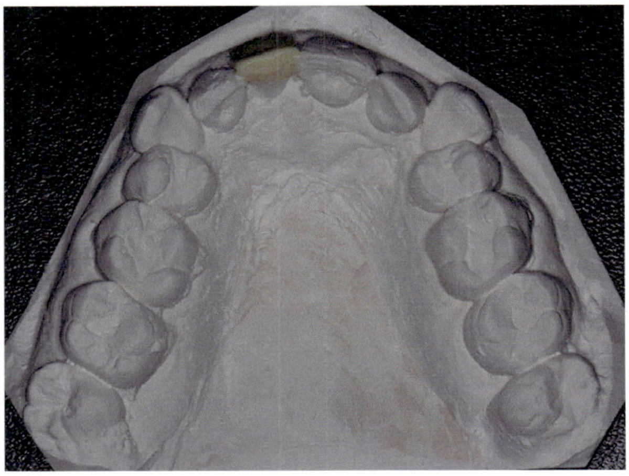

FIGURE 168c

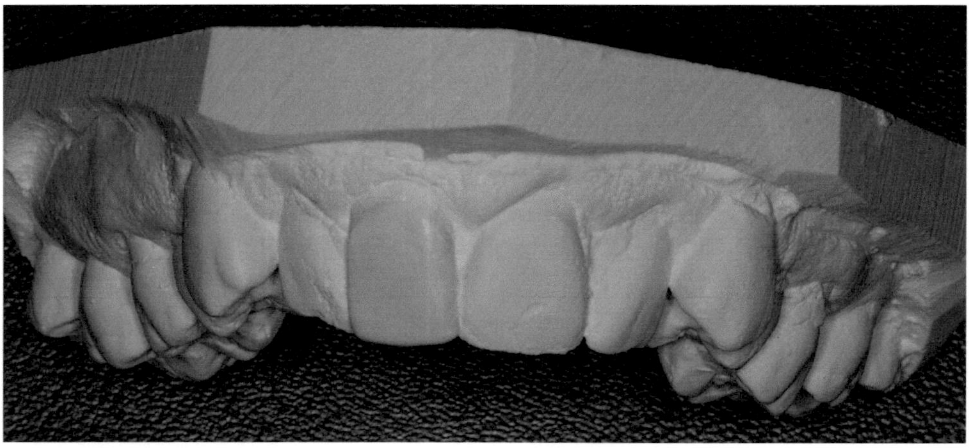

The patient in ***Figure 168*** came in because he wanted to correct the upper right tooth, which was very proclined. I recommended orthodontic treatment, but he didn't want to go through with it.

To show him how much tooth reduction would be needed, I carried out a wax up and showed him how it would look. Even if a lot of tooth reduction was to take place, the shape of the two central incisors was never going to be the same due to a lack of space (***Figure 168c***).

Eventually the patient agreed to have orthodontic treatment to get the right aesthetic. Yet he was an example of how a patient might sometimes need some extra help to understand why they need braces.

Before/midway/after photos

Of course, whenever a patient agrees to your treatment (e.g. ***Figure 169a***), they might still be nursing doubts in the back of their mind. Mid-treatment photos are the perfect tool for ridding them of that doubt.

Therefore take mid-treatment photos (***Figure 169b***) after removal of all the restorations. Sometimes it's worth leaving the caries and taking photos, before complete removal, showing them to the patient and highlighting how much decay there was beneath their old restoration.

Afterwards take a post-treatment photo (***Figure 169c***) and sit down with the patient, showing them how the treatment went and what was done.

FIGURE 169a

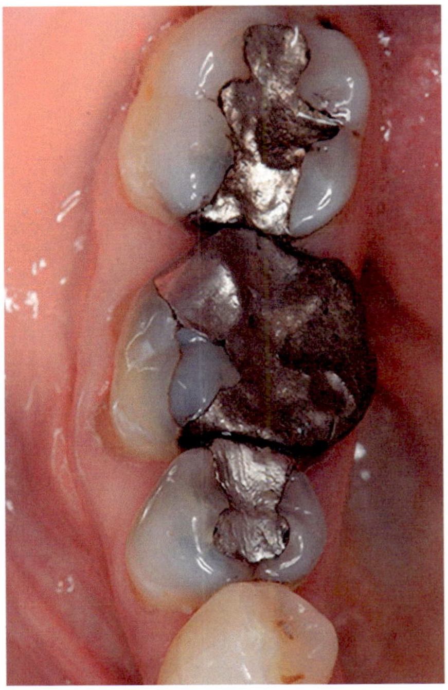

FIGURE 169b

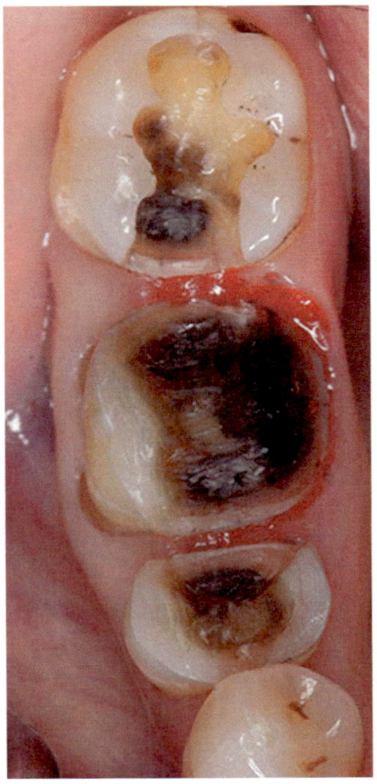

FIGURE 169c

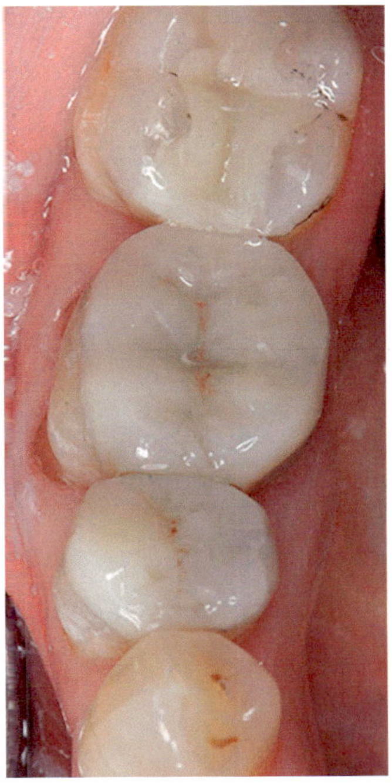

Such an educational tool is very helpful. This is because next time you recommend that a patient undergoes treatment, they will be less likely to doubt you, based on what you have done for them in the past.

Before and after

Before (***Figure 170a***) and after (***Figure 170b***) photos are crucial when you're showing the patient a full mouth reconstruction case, as they need to visualise how their teeth will look after you're finished up with treatment. The best way to achieve this is by showing the patient similar cases you've treated in the past.

FIGURE 170a

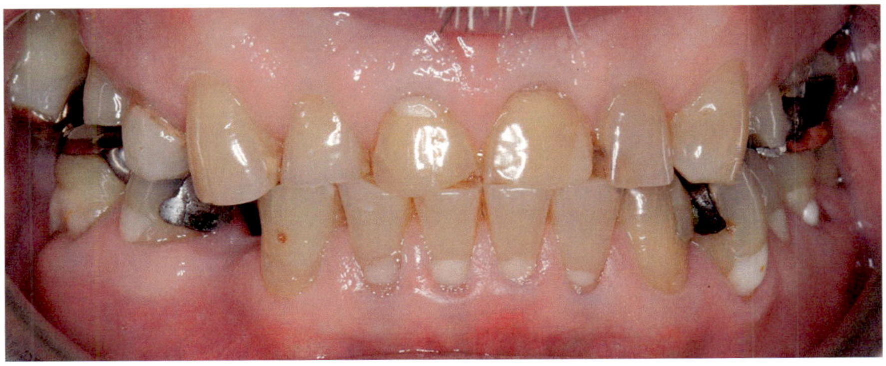

FIGURE 170b

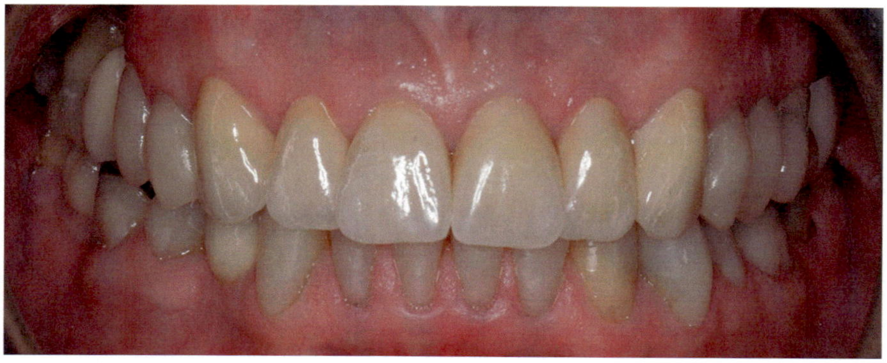

Of course, you can do a digital mock-up as that also gives patients some perspective. But showing patients before and after photos of your previous patients will help them understand that you have done these cases before and that you're capable of helping them reach their goals.

Top tips

Let us look at some important aspects of communication.

Building rapport:

- When doing an examination I change my tone of voice. If it's monotonous and not going high or low, then the patient may lose interest. Therefore, make sure you change your tone of voice depending on whether you want to emphasise some of the words, increase the tonality of the voice to make an impact. If you are concerned about something, then you lower your voice as you explain it to the patient.
- Make sure you listen attentively to the patient. Many times, we listen to respond, but make sure you just listen without aiming to respond right away. Make sure you have a nurse who is recording what the patient is saying so that you don't have to think about writing things down. I still have a notepad for writing down important points about what the patient is saying. But when you're writing in the notepad, patients get distracted and may lose your train of thought. Therefore, make sure you listen and have someone else take notes for you.
- Ask questions. I ask lots of questions before I give any solution, as I really need to know exactly what the patient is looking for and what problems they are suffering from.
- Make sure you find out the patient's goal before you plan any treatment, and try to encourage them to consider long-term goals and visions rather than short-term ones. Often patients will prefer immediate goals, such as trying to save money by doing

short-term treatment rather than looking at the long-term, and hoping to save that money right now compared to spending the money and making sure the treatment lasts longer.

- Once you've talked, summarise everything back to the patient. It's best to repeat the patient's problems in their own words to make sure you have understood them correctly.

Examination:

- Do a comprehensive examination for each patient that sees you. They need to feel that you're taking the time and that you care.
- Whenever you're doing any comprehensive examination, dictate the state of the tooth to your nurse. If you mention details, e.g. an upper right second molar has a large amalgam restoration, a leaking amalgam restoration, crack line on the mesial aspect, caries around the restoration and an open margin, then the patient is also paying attention as to what they have in their mouth.
- Furthermore, announcing non findings such as negative results for cancer or gum disease really builds trust, as patients know that you are doing a thorough assessment. If there are lots of problems then the patient must also be made aware of this.
- As a result, whenever I'm finished with an examination it will be common for a patient to acknowledge the problem their mouth has. Again, you are trying to eliminate doubt from the patient's mind by making them understand that you are assessing everything.
- With all my checkups, even the routine ones, I always take five photographs: 1) front smile, 2) retracted view with close, 3) retracted view open 4) occlusal upper 5) occlusal lower. These photographs are very important for patient communication.

Discussion of current situation:

- Once I've done the examination, I will then sit down with the patient and show them each and every tooth on the photographs I've taken, explaining the findings.
- Make sure that you show the patient these photos even if they don't have a complaint or even if you haven't found anything. If a patient has got good teeth, take photos and make them feel happy that they have nothing wrong with their teeth. They will be grateful that you have taken the time to explain to them that there is nothing wrong with their teeth.

Discussion of treatment options:

- When it comes to doing treatment planning, make sure that you create some options. Think about what the patient wants and the issues you have recorded when you're building the rapport.

- Make sure you plan and propose treatment that is in line with their issues, goals and demands.
- Give a recommendation. Often dentists are reluctant to do this. Many don't want to make patients feel obliged or pressured into having treatment done. Yet giving recommendation is very important because the patient is coming to you for an expert opinion on their mouth. Unless you give the patient a sense of what you think is the best choice, the patient will have four or five options and get confused, most likely resulting in them not having any treatment done.

So, make sure you're articulating what you think is best for them while at the same time telling the patient that you're prepared to do whatever they want you to do, out of the options you have proposed. You need to make sure that they know which option is best in light of their situation, long-term goals, and needs.

- When giving patients options, follow this format: tell them what you're offering, what it means, and how it will benefit them. Eg. say to them that they need an implant to replace a missing tooth, which is a fixed option which means they will be able to chew food without having to worry about putting something in and taking it out, or whatever the patient's worry is. You therefore align that worry or issue with your proposed treatment plan.

Fees:

- When it comes to discussing fees, make sure you have set fees for almost everything. This helps to avoid any misunderstandings the patient might have. So, make sure that you clarify what the fees are for composites, onlays, zirconia or porcelain crowns, etc.
- There will be some fees which inevitably are not set in stone. However, write all the fees down so that your nurses know and it's there on the computer or in your record. So, whenever you're planning the fees, go straight to your notes so that you're not having to re-think and potentially reduce your prices.
- Sometimes if you are doing a treatment and you don't know what the fee is going to be because, for example, you haven't removed a crown yet, tell the patient that you don't know what lies underneath that crown until it's removed. The situation is hard to know until then. If you can save the tooth, then you will do the new crown at a certain price. If the tooth needs to come out, then the removal and replacement will be at a certain price. In short, make it clear to them that these are the options and these are the prices.

General:

- Make sure when you're doing an assessment or a discussion with the patient that you do not clock watch, for your next patient. You need to accept that when you take time, you will run late.
- You will get rejected. Sometimes I'll spend an hour discussing a treatment plan with a patient, only to have them say that they don't want it. You need to be able to take that on the chin, and don't get upset because at the end of the day, you're trying to help them. If they do not accept your help, then it's their loss, not yours.
- You might think that you're trying to sell something. But again, as I said, whenever you are doing any treatment planning, keep in mind that you're trying to help the patient - not simply selling something to them.

The two-appointment system

I've been asked many times whether to do two appointments or propose the treatment plan during the first appointment. The answer is that it really depends.

- **Multiple issues but lack of time to explain**
  If a patient comes to me with a very complex treatment, I won't propose the treatment plan on the same appointment. Instead, I will stop after telling them what they have in their mouth and call the patient back again so I can assess the information and plan treatment. However, if the patient is really keen then I will be happy to give them some ideas.

- **Change in OVD**
  Similarly, if I'm changing the patient's OVD then that means it's a full mouth reconstruction case. Obviously, even if I'm calling a patient back, I will give them some rough estimate as to how much it will all be as I want to see whether the patient can afford that treatment.

  If a patient cannot afford the treatment, there's no point in continuing. However, if you have created enough value then there is a good chance that the patient may accept your plan.

- **Aesthetic cases and Implants**
  Aesthetic cases or even complex implants will need some more planning. That's why if it's a single implant then the system I've outlined can be very good.

  I've recorded videos for patients and sent them before they come to see me and hence I would ideally have answered almost every question they can imagine on those videos.

When they come in, I'll have a look at their mouth. If it's a single implant and they know exactly what the fees are then they'll hopefully understand the process, ensuring that communicating with them will be easier.

However, if it's a complex case involving a full mouth implant, then I'll usually schedule two appointments because I need to really understand what's going on in their mouth by taking some radiographs, maybe do a CBCT scan, and see them again.

Money issues for dentists

Many dentists underestimate the value of the work they do. This is a self limiting belief, which makes many dentists uncomfortable proposing high value treatment. They feel that their treatment is not worth the money they charge. This holds them back from proposing the treatment. We desire to please our patients and make them happy by not charging them too much money. This results in dentists undercharging patients.

This is another reason many dentists would rather not do full mouth reconstruction or other expensive treatment. We avoid offering the best treatment to avoid causing short term upset to our patients and discomfort to ourselves. However, this approach fails to do the patient justice, denying them the information they have come to a dentist to get and denying them the ability to make an informed decision.

The patients come to you to get a professional opinion or advice on their oral health and their options. If you're not telling them what's going on in their mouth and the best option, in your opinion, for them out of all the available options, then it's just not fair. It is paternalistic to make financial decisions on behalf of the patient. The decision should be theirs, your job is to enable them to make an informed decision.

I would advise you to make sure that you give the patient all the details irrespective of the patient's financial status. It is your job to tell exactly what they have in their mouth. Whether they can afford it or not is beyond your control. Your job is to be honest with your patients and clearly explain what the treatment options are and which option is best for them, in your professional opinion.

Fees

Whenever it comes to fees, patients will have almost one of these four concerns.

- **They can't afford it all at once.** If this is the concern, then you need to have finance options available. This means they can spread the cost of the treatment over multiple months or years in installments they can afford.
- **A patient says that the same treatment is cheaper somewhere else.** Explain why you are offering them expensive treatment. To do this you need to make sure you build enough value into your treatment during communication, discussions and rapport building with your patient. If a patient says the same treatment is cheaper elsewhere, then you haven't shown that patient why you're charging what you're charging. Usually, this is the reason they are coming up with this kind of statement.
- **Patients feel they don't understand why the treatment is so expensive.** Again, this is the reason you need to build value into your treatment. You need to help them understand: explain the process, how long it takes, how many hours you will be spending on their teeth, and what these hours involve. You need to explain just how many people are involved in the process: the technician, the digital technician, you, your nurses. The patient should know how many appointments it will take, and exactly what you and your entire team are going to do in each appointment. It is best practice to clearly address all these questions before the patient asks them. Otherwise, it can look like you are making excuses. So, build the value first, through explaining to your patient just how much work you will be doing for them before even they ask these questions.
- **Sometimes, the patient genuinely cannot afford it.** As I said, before patients in this category are much less common than we tend to believe. Most of the time, when patients claim that they can't afford it, this means that they haven't seen the value in what you're offering. And as a clinician it's our job to communicate that value.

Diagnosis

There are often serious issues with diagnosis which result in patients getting insufficient treatment. Underdiagnosis is more of an issue than overdiagnosis from what I have seen.

I see patients coming into the dental surgery where I work, and a colleague sends me photos, in my opinion full mouth reconstruction is needed for that patient. However, sometimes a colleague's plan is just to build front six teeth and maybe do a DAHL in the patient's mouth. However, what I see is that the patient needs full mouth reconstruction because their posterior teeth are worn, they're heavily filled, and they really need that treatment. But sometimes dentists just can't seem to make that jump from just anterior teeth to full mouth reconstruction. They end up under diagnosing their patient.

Again, no diagnosis is an issue for patients with mild tooth wear or mild to moderate tooth wear. Of course, if it's a severe tooth wear, dentists will notice it, and they will be able to identify, and tell patients. However, mild to moderate tooth wear, which is very common, routinely gets ignored.

Treatment plan

When it comes to doing treatment, very often, dentists offer no treatment and monitoring of the mild to moderate tooth wear. We know that when the dentine is exposed, it will continue to wear down, so we must offer some sort of treatment, for example, protective or preventative treatment.

We discussed previously that very often, dentists plan the treatment which is based on their underdiagnosis and based on their current skills. This is because they lack the confidence to prepare a comprehensive treatment plan.

Underpromising and overdelivering

Having said all this, when you are proposing treatment to your patient, make sure you underpromise and overdeliver rather than overpromise and underdeliver.

The scenario where you have overpromised and underdelivered is usually the result of poor communication. Because the patient did not understand exactly what they were getting and you did not communicate well enough for the patient to understand why they got what they got. It is also possible that you were not yet skilled enough to provide the promised treatment. So the end result does not match your promise.

Specific tips for full mouth reconstruction cases

- Make sure you give patients some rough prices after you have built up rapport and communicated enough value in the first appointment. In some cases, the patient just does not see, even if you communicate perfectly and do everything to build up the value. If they do not see why they need to invest into their health, then another appointment would be a waste of both your and their time. Give them a rough estimate, a rough idea. By going through this whole book, perhaps several times if needed, you will have learned to do this quickly. Let the patient know the price range. If then they say they can't afford it, then there is no point in taking their case further. Of course, you give patients different options which are within their budget range. But if it's a full mouth construction, and they say they can't afford it, then you can't do the treatment and there's no point in calling them back.

- Make sure you have your finance options ready.
- Always send patients pre-consultation information including the appropriate videos. This is especially important for implant cases where there's a lot to take in, where the patient may not be able to understand everything during the consultation. It is wise to establish commitment during the first consultation. So, give them all the information they need before they come and see you. Then, they are fully prepared.
- Always show the patient before and after cases to build your rapport, communicate and build your value and show them what is achievable. Make sure that you don't forget to show them the testimonials of previous patients.
- Last but not least, make this a team effort. Your whole team should be involved in the communication process in order to give the best chance of success. Otherwise, the patient does not see their treatment as a team effort. If the patient walks in and the receptionist is not welcoming and perhaps even rude to them, or if the nurse doesn't take part in the conversation, then your patient may not feel that they will be well looked after. So make sure your whole team coordinates and is involved in the process.

Although I have given you an overview of communication here, I encourage you to join our online course to get more information.

By enrolling into my Online *Practical Guide to Full Mouth Reconstruction Book* Course using code 'fmrbook' you will get access not only to the FMR course, but also to the free communication course that comes with it.

Scan the QR code below to access it:

As usual, if you are having any issues accessing the link by using the QR code, then do not hesitate to contact me at https://drdevangpatel.com/contact/.

I hope you found this textbook helpful. Congratulations on finishing this book and I hope you have all the information needed to carry out your first direct adhesive full mouth reconstruction case. By this point you may already find that you have enough information to carry out direct adhesive full mouth reconstruction cases, to price them correctly and to communicate with patients to create win-win situations, or you may find that you have everything you need after you enroll into the online course, so make sure you do that as well.

If you have any questions, please feel free to contact me via filling out the webform at www.drdevangpate.com and I'll do everything I can to help you. Also remember that this book is LIVE which means that you will get updates on any changes as long as you have registered.

References

Banerji, S., Mehta, S., Opdam, N., Loomans, B. (2020) Practical Procedures in the Management of Tooth Wear.

Dawson, P. (2006) Functional Occlusion From TMJ to Smile Design, Hardback.

Nelson, S. DDS MS (2020) Wheeler's Dental Anatomy, Physiology and Occlusion.

Magne, P. (2021) Biomimetic Restorative Dentistry.

Okeson, J., Management of Temporomandibular Disorders and Occlusion. 8th Edition.

Pameijer, J. H.N. (1983) Periodontal and Occlusal Factors in Crown and Bridge Procedures. Chapter 5.

Wassel, R., Naru, A., Steel, J., Nohl F. (2008 Applied Occlusion (Quintessentials of Dental Practice).

"Combining traditional and adhesive dentistry to reconstruct the excessively worn dentition". European Journal of Aesthetic Dentistry. 2008, Vol 3, No 3, 270-289.

Posselt, U. (1952). Studies in the mobility of the mandible, Acta Odontologica Scandinavica, 10 (Supplement), 1–160.

Shupe RJ., Mohamed SE., Christensen LV.,Finger IM., Weinberg R. (1984) Effects of Occlusal guidance on Jaw Muscle Activity. Journal of Prosthetic Dentistry. 51(6):811.

Standlee JP., Caputo AA., Ralph JP. (1979) Stress Transfer to the Mandible during Anterior Guidance and Group Function Eccentric Movements.. Journal of Prosthetic Dentistry. 41(1):35-9.

Made in the USA
Las Vegas, NV
03 November 2026

57422772R00152